Prepping
for a
Pandemic

Lifesaving Supplies, Skills and Plans for Surviving an Outbreak

Cat Ellis

ULYSSES PRESS

This book is dedicated to every reader and audience member who e-mailed me with questions about pandemics.
This is for you.

✳ ✳ ✳

Published in the US by:
Ulysses Press
P.O. Box 3440
Berkeley, CA 94703
www.ulyssespress.com

ISBN: 978-1-61243-451-3
Library of Congress Control Number: 2015937575

Printed in Canada by Marquis Book Printing

10 9 8 7 6 5 4 3 2

Acquisitions editor: Kelly Reed
Project editor: Casie Vogel
Managing editor: Claire Chun
Editor: Paula Dragosh
Proofreader: Renee Rutledge
Design and layout: what!design @ whatweb.com
Cover artwork: female © swissmacky/shutterstock.com, grunge texture
    © Alexey Pushkin/shutterstock.com
Index: Sayre Van Young

Contents

Foreword:
Deadly Disease and Disaster Go Hand in Hand

Many of us believe that the possibility of a deadly pandemic occurring is implausible. After all, we live in an advanced society where we are witnessing some of the greatest medical achievements in history. But all the medical breakthroughs in the world will not prepare us for dealing with a large-scale pandemic. This type of natural disaster is longer lasting and harder felt than most and is both volatile and devastating in its own right.

It's a big gamble to think that we're immune from this type of disaster reaching us. It wasn't that long ago that the 1918 Spanish flu hit with such force that it tested every parameter of life as we knew it. The Spanish flu came in three waves and was called the "greatest medical holocaust in history." As *The Prepper's Blueprint* explains:

> because of a rare shift of genetic material in the virus, no one had been able to build an immunity to the virus. The death toll was estimated at between 30 million and 50 million people worldwide. It moved so fast that within the first 6 months, 25 million people had caught the Spanish Flu. More people died in one year of this flu than in the entire 4 years of the medieval Black Plague. By turning into a vicious form of pneumonia, this strain of influenza killed people, often within hours of the first signs of illness. . . . So many people died at once that there was

a shortage of morticians, coffins and gravediggers. Morgues were forced to stack bodies like "cordwood" in the hallways and mass graves were dug to try and deal with all of the corpses in an effort to prevent even more health risks. Public health ordinances were created to try to contain the pandemic, to little avail.

It's not far-fetched to think that we could once again see another outbreak like this. In fact, many scientists believe that it's just a matter of time before history repeats itself. Illnesses once considered eradicated are beginning to show signs of life again. This could be because of our population-dense communities and ease in transportation. In 2015 visitors at Disneyland found themselves exposed to measles that most likely originated in the Philippines.

In this day and age, we must expect the unexpected and accept that if we were to face a crisis in which medications, sanitation, and other modern standards and resources were unavailable, these deadly diseases would quickly spread and have the capacity to cause a devastating disaster the world has not seen for a century.

In this indispensable book, Cat Ellis explains how quickly a pandemic emergency can overwhelm a community by exposing cracks in how unprepared our hospitals are for handling highly infectious diseases, how our transportation systems will be shut down, and how quickly a frightened population can descend into acts of crime and violence. As unsettling as this sounds, it only emphasizes the importance of having your own personal plan for survival.

We must keep in mind that we're never safe from bacteria, viruses, and diseases, but we can prepare accordingly. Cat points out that to better prepare for pandemics, we must understand the diseases in question: how they communicate and how they survive in nature. Only then can we find the answers we need to protect ourselves. In this book, she lists the diseases likely to spread after a disaster, and actionable steps to take in your preparedness planning.

Cat Ellis and I share a common appreciation for natural remedies. In her first book, *Prepper's Natural Medicine*, she asks the reader point-blank, "What would you do if there were no pharmacy?" In a postdisaster event, we may not have access to pharmacies, hospitals, and modern medical care. Her focus on herbal remedies creates a balanced and layered medical approach that should be part of any well-rounded preparedness plan. This is what I believe sets this book apart from other pandemic manuals.

Deadly diseases and disasters go hand in hand. This book helps you understand the many overarching themes that emerge in the discussion of pandemic preparedness and shows you ways to get ready for each one. In a time of uncertainty, equipping yourself with knowledge and the necessary tools needed to survive a pandemic will keep you and your family ahead of the problem. Cat says it perfectly in the book, "Pandemics will happen. When, where, what, for how long, and how bad will it be? I don't know. No one knows. What I do know, however, is that being prepared means that you and your loved ones stand a greater chance of surviving something as devastating and as drawn out as a pandemic."

TESS PENNINGTON
Founder, Ready Nutrition, and the author of *The Prepper's Cookbook* and *The Prepper's Blueprint*

Preface

Ever since I started my website, www.HerbalPrepper.com, I have been fortunate to have an active, engaging, and inquisitive readership and podcast audience. My readers and listeners never fail to push me to investigate more and look into scenarios I might not have considered. To get their questions answered, I have had to leave my comfort zone as an herbalist and reach out to doctors, nurses, EMTs, and former combat medics to find answers. I have spent untold hours reading medical studies on various illnesses and conventional treatments, and seeking out evidence-based alternatives. I am a better herbalist today because of my audience and the friendships forged with the mainstream medical field.

While I was working on my first book, *Prepper's Natural Medicine: Lifesaving Herbs, Essential Oils, and Natural Remedies for When There Is No Doctor*, the media was focused on outbreaks of two deadly diseases. The first was Middle East respiratory syndrome (MERS), a new, viral, respiratory infection with the potential for respiratory failure and a high mortality rate. It was especially deadly if the patient also suffered from a chronic illness, with diabetics having the highest risk of death.

MERS was a new disease, one that humans had never encountered before and therefore had no prior exposure or immunity to. Eventually, a doctor working in Saudi Arabia contracted the virus and got on a plane to the United States, where he attended a medical conference. Within days, another traveler came from Saudi Arabia to Florida, and that person was diagnosed with MERS. While these exposures to the deadly MERS virus were contained, they were a wake-up call for all Americans that in our modern world, the next outbreak may be only one plane ride away.

The second outbreak developed in West Africa. It was an Ebola outbreak, the likes of which no one had ever seen. Instead of burning through victims in remote villages, Ebola took hold in crowded, poverty-stricken cities with transportation links. This, plus border permeability, led to Ebola passing from Guinea to Sierra Leone to Liberia. New infections continue to cross and recross the borders, reinfecting previously cleared areas.

After our brush with MERS, surely we were ready for Ebola. Unfortunately, we were not. A man from West Africa traveled to Dallas, Texas, and began to exhibit symptoms. After initially being misdiagnosed with the flu and sent home, the man returned to the hospital and was correctly diagnosed with Ebola. We were told the virus spread to two nurses.

When I wasn't working, I was glued to my television and Internet, waiting to hear or read the latest information on either outbreak. I cataloged article after article on both MERS and Ebola. Naturally, a high percentage of the e-mails from my audience was about these diseases and what to do in the event of a pandemic. What was the real risk of either? If Ebola came here, would it be as virulent, since our climate and environment are nothing like Africa? Our most elite hospitals could handle a few Ebola patients, but what about the local hospitals? Were protocols even in place to deal with either MERS or Ebola?

I set out to answer these questions for my readers and listeners. I looked at conventional treatments and herbal treatments of related illnesses. For example, while MERS was a new coronavirus, herbal medicines had been used successfully in another coronavirus that attacked the respiratory system, severe acute respiratory syndrome (SARS). While there's no guarantee that the same herbs would be effective for MERS, it's a good place from which to make a hypothesis and come up with a backup plan.

With Ebola, there's no cure. There's no drug, vaccine, or natural remedy. But the conventional approach of keeping the patient hydrated adequately to prevent the organ failure and shock common to Ebola fatalities goes a long way to saving that patient. This was encouraging, but Ebola was still contagious, seemingly even with loads of personal protective equipment (PPE). This led me to research the types of PPE being used, noting their differences and vulnerabilities during the decontamination process when removing PPE. The best suits are prohibitively expensive for the average person, but what, if anything, could be assembled that would provide the same level of protection? If such PPE could be assembled affordably, then it could be used for any pandemic, especially of unknown and new diseases.

Antibiotic resistance is one of several reasons I started my website. This is a viable threat, one we will all have to deal with, and we need alternatives now. There are several bacterial infections on this list because they can be fatal and have demonstrated resistance to antibiotic drugs. Some of these bacteria have strains that have already adapted and developed resistance to all known antibiotics. It's only a matter of time before the other strains develop total drug resistance. We must have other options: soon, we'll have a serious problem, including the potential for a pandemic.

I decided to take all the information that I had gathered and compile it into a single resource on what happens during a pandemic, not just with a specific illness, but also the routes of disease in transmission, how to protect against transmission, and what to expect from the authorities. What is the media's role, what are the government's priorities, and what are steps we take to protect our families from the pandemic illness itself while maintaining security over the supplies and resources we'll need during such a disaster?

Sometimes, things don't work out the way we plan. Sometimes, there's no good answer or solution. Sometimes, there has to be some speculation and educated guessing. I've tried to blend the best of evidence-based approaches with some measure of speculation when necessary to arrive at what I consider the top seven threats for the next great pandemic, and an appropriate response. The research and creation of this book have been an important exercise for me to improve my own family's level of preparedness, as well as fulfill the obligation to my audience to get these questions answered to the best of my ability. I hope that you, the reader, find it useful.

CHAPTER 1

A Learning Moment:
2014's Deadly Ebola Outbreak

The 2014 Ebola pandemic is both a sad and ongoing catastrophe, as well as an important lesson. This outbreak has claimed more lives and lasted longer than any other Ebola outbreak. It has also provided the world with an opportunity to see what a deadly pandemic looks like and what kind of global response, or lack thereof, we can expect.

What we have seen is not good. We are poorly prepared to face such an event, both as individuals and as a nation. While this outbreak is an enormous tragedy, not learning the lessons of it would be an even greater tragedy.

The Beginnings of a Pandemic

The Ebola crisis, which officially began in December 2013, originated in the West African nation of Guinea and quickly spread to nearby Liberia and Sierra Leone. Past outbreaks had always proved so deadly that they would burn themselves out quickly. But that's not what happened this time.

This time, instead of starting in some dark and remote part of the central African jungle, far removed from civilization, this outbreak began in a small village in Guinea, Meliandou. While Meliandou is small, it is not far from larger populations.

Unfortunately, no one recognized the early cases as Ebola. Other severe illnesses, such as cholera and malaria, which share many of the same initial symptoms as the highly infectious Ebola, are endemic to the area. Ebola spread easily to family members and caregivers. Patients began to show up at the hospital in nearby Guéckédou, and still the true cause was not recognized.

It may seem strange that Ebola was initially misdiagnosed as cholera or malaria. These diseases, however, are so prevalent in this area that seven of the early patients tested positive for cholera even though their symptoms were not exactly like cholera. Like something out of a nightmare, these poor people had both cholera and Ebola at the same time. It also meant that Ebola was permitted to fly under the radar undetected just a little longer.

Fortunately, Médecins Sans Frontières (Doctors Without Borders) was already in the area responding to a malaria outbreak. The volunteer medical organization stepped in to help support the local doctors with what they believed was a cholera outbreak. But three months into this supposed outbreak, only one thing was clear: this was not cholera.

In mid-March 2014, at its Geneva office, Doctors Without Borders in Guinea consulted with a "disease detective" who suggested it was a hemorrhagic fever, either Marburg or Ebola. Guinea's Ministry of Health then sent samples out for testing. When test results came back from Paris confirming the pathogen to be Ebola Zaire, the most deadly known strain of Ebola, everything changed.

Local doctors and hospitals were soon overwhelmed. Doctors Without Borders became the primary source of Ebola care to the region. On March 23, 2014, supplies of PPE were dispatched by the World Health Organization (WHO) to Conakry, Guinea's capital, largest city, and transportation hub. It was a mere four days later, on March 27, 2014, when Conakry saw its own first Ebola patients, and there were more popping up in the surrounding area. It wasn't long before cases were found in Sierra Leone and Liberia. It's suspected that border permeability assisted movement through these countries, allowing for resurgences of Ebola weeks and months after an area had been declared clear.

Public Reaction

In the United States, the Ebola outbreak initially got little more than a raised eyebrow from most people. It was half a world away. It was depressing, but not our problem. In the beginning of the outbreak, the media gave it the standard treatment, minimal coverage with feigned concern and compassion. But in the coming months, the story took over the news. It gave the media everything they could want to drive ratings: drama, death, anguish, and the potential threat that this deadly disease might come here.

The local populations of Guinea, Sierra Leone, and Liberia, however, did not have the luxury of ignoring the outbreak. They were devastated and suffering. They were also fearful of the foreign health care workers and Ebola clinics. Their loved ones went in but didn't come out. People were not permitted to conduct their traditional funerary and burial rituals. The health care workers were dressed unlike any other health care workers they had ever seen, covered head to toe in protective gear.

Information often calms fears. But in this case, there was little information. How did this happen? How did this virus, which had never been seen outside a very different and distant part of the continent, end up in West Africa? How did the first person in the outbreak get infected? We just don't know.

This vacuum of information led to the local populations filling in the blanks on their own. Suspicion, rumors, and mistrust brewed among the locals. They began to blame the very volunteers who had come to help them for causing the disease and the deaths. Family members tried to hide and care for loved ones at home rather than risk them dying in the clinics where burial rituals would be denied. Predictably, this only helped spread both the disease and the fear.

The first attack on a volunteer Ebola clinic happened in early April in Guinea. On April 4, 2014, two local mobs attacked a clinic, claiming that Doctors Without Borders had brought Ebola to the area. The medical team serving the community had to be evacuated and the clinic was abandoned. It would not be the last attack.

On August 17, 2014, one of the most brazen attacks on an Ebola observation clinic took place in the slum area of West Point, Liberia. Fueled by fear of Ebola, foreign health care workers, and preexisting mistrust of the government, a team of armed men stormed a clinic, claiming to be "liberating" the twenty-nine Ebola patients inside. The men chanted "No Ebola in West Point!" They looted the clinic and stole contaminated medical equipment and bloodstained mattresses and bed linens.

Not only was this a threat to those who came in contact with the contaminated supplies, but it also raised concerns about the potential for terrorists to come into possession of these items. What could a terrorist do with such things? Could contaminated materials, such as bed linens and IV supplies, be used to spread Ebola in an attack? Would that be possible?

This came on the heels of the Centers for Disease Control and Prevention (CDC) issuing new recommendations to airlines for cleaning their cabins between flights, prohibiting the use of pressurized air. The pressurized air posed a risk of temporarily sending the virus airborne. This inspired a rumor that CDC was worried that Ebola had mutated and gone airborne.

Ebola in the United States

On August 7, 2014, CDC director Tom Frieden testified to the Committee of Foreign Affairs that it was "inevitable" that international travelers would arrive in the United States after visiting the affected region and would have symptoms. Here's the full quote from the transcript:

> It is the first time we are having to deal with it here in the United States, and that is not merely because of the two people who became ill caring for Ebola patients and were brought back to the U.S. by their organization. That is primarily because we are all connected, and inevitably there will be travelers,

American citizens and others, who go from these three countries, or from Lagos, if it doesn't get it under control, and are here with symptoms. Those symptoms might be Ebola or something else. So we are having to deal with Ebola in the US in a way that we have never had to deal with it before.[1]

Headlines on mainstream and alternative media alike stated in big, bold letters that the CDC director testified that the spread of Ebola to the United States was "inevitable" because of modern air travel. Even though that's not exactly what he said, Ebola's inevitable spread to the United States was the more attention-grabbing story. Conspiracy theories were already running wild here in the United States, and Director Frieden's comments were like pouring gasoline on a fire.

Just a few days before the director testified, two Americans who contracted Ebola while volunteering to care for Ebola patients in West Africa were evacuated to the United States for treatment in Atlanta. Having Ebola much closer to home was alarming. People wondered if the government was being too casual about the risk, or even if the government would risk such an outbreak intentionally. Others saw the risk as minimal and judged those with concerns as being heartless and alarmist. Ebola was proving to be just as divisive as every other media story.

Both patients brought to Atlanta from Liberia survived. One was a physician, Dr. Kent Brantly, who received a blood transfusion from a patient who recovered from Ebola under his care. The other was a volunteer, Nancy Writebol, who was working in Liberia decontaminating health care workers who were treating Ebola patients. Both Brantly and Writebol received an experimental drug called ZMapp.

A third patient, Dr. Rick Sacra, was evacuated from Liberia to Nebraska, where he received an experimental treatment, as well as a blood transfusion from Dr. Brantly. Sacra also survived. He had been working in Liberia for years volunteering in a maternity ward and was not there as an Ebola volunteer. Another patient evacuated from Sierra Leone to Atlanta in September was in the hospital for a month,

---

1   http://docs.house.gov/meetings/FA/FA16/20140807/102607/HHRG-113-FA16-Transcript-20140807.pdf.

recovered, and was discharged. That patient has chosen to remain anonymous, and all that's known is that the patient worked for WHO.

Amid the fear, there seemed to be some hope for treatment. After all, the United States had now successfully treated three Ebola patients on US soil. With the length of this outbreak, doctors finally had a chance to see what care was most effective to help people survive long enough to fight the virus off on their own. Transfusions from those who survived helped, as did keeping patients as hydrated as possible.

The First Victim in the United States

And then, it happened. A man in Texas who came to the United States from Liberia to visit family here, Thomas Eric Duncan, was brought to the hospital by ambulance and later tested positive for Ebola.

There was anger and fear over what seemed to be Director Frieden's warning come true. A person did indeed travel to the United States by plane and bring the Ebola virus. There was all manner of speculation on whether Duncan knew that he was ill before coming to the United States or whether he developed symptoms here. Were the safety protocols for screening passengers sufficient or even followed in Duncan's case?

Any good feelings that people may have had about our ability to meet the challenge of Ebola went out the window with Duncan's case. Duncan did not get to go to an elite facility, such as Atlanta or Nebraska. Instead, Duncan went to his local hospital, Texas Health Presbyterian Hospital in Dallas, just like any of us would. At each step along the way, his case was mishandled, resulting in his death and the spread of Ebola to two nurses who selflessly cared for him.

The mistakes started with his first visit to the hospital. Duncan went to the emergency room on September 25, 2014, with a fever, abdominal pain, dizziness, nausea, and headache. Obtaining his recent travel information was not part of the emergency room's intake process, and he was sent back to the waiting room.

When Duncan was finally seen in the emergency room, a nurse documented his symptoms as sharp, intermittent epigastric and upper abdominal pain. She noted that he was from Africa, but not where in Africa. This information was not communicated verbally to the doctor but written into Duncan's file.

When the physician finally saw Duncan, the official record shows that the doctor directly interviewed him and his companion (girlfriend). The medical records state that Duncan was a local resident and had not been around sick people, nor did he have any nausea, vomiting, or diarrhea. After doing routine lab work, the doctor made a diagnosis of sinusitis with abdominal pain. He was sent home the following morning with an informational sheet on sinus infections and told to drink lots of fluids and rest.

Duncan returned to the apartment he was sharing with his relatives and remained there. His condition worsened. On September 28, 2014, he went by ambulance back to Texas Health Presbyterian Hospital with fever, abdominal pain, and diarrhea. This time, the physician was alert, noted that Duncan had recently come from Liberia, ordered that the patient be tested for Ebola, and initiated strict CDC protocols for treating an Ebola patient. Duncan, who had developed explosive diarrhea and projectile vomiting, was moved to an intensive care unit that was emptied of all other patients to create a makeshift isolation unit.

Here we had an individual who had recently come from a country with an active Ebola outbreak who brought himself to the emergency room when he started showing symptoms. He sat in a waiting room with other patients without any kind of barrier or protection against infection and was initially sent home to live in close contact with his family.

Once Duncan was admitted on his second trip to the emergency room, the family was quarantined in the same apartment with Duncan's contaminated bed linens and belongings. How he did not spread the disease to his relatives, and then they spread it to the larger community, is nothing short of a miracle.

These were the kinds of scenarios that authorities had repeatedly reassured the public couldn't possibly happen. Yet they did. Duncan died on October 8, 2014.

Quarantine and Protocol Failure

During his final days, Duncan was treated by more than seventy dedicated staff members, including two nurses who somehow became infected with the deadly Ebola virus even though they were wearing the personal protective equipment provided by the hospital. But the PPE these nurses wore had open necks, instead of gear that completely covered their entire bodies.

Nurse Nina Pham, who provided care for Duncan in his last days, became ill just days after Duncan's death. On October 12, 2014, she tested positive for Ebola and was put in isolation and sent to a National Institutes of Health hospital in Maryland for treatment. Two days after Pham tested positive, a second nurse who treated Duncan, Amber Joy Vinson, developed a fever. She was isolated and the next day got her test results back confirming that she, too, had Ebola.

Officials from CDC, including Director Frieden, took an unexpected position, blaming the nurses for not properly following protocols. This blame game didn't sit well with many, including the nurse's union, which spoke out on the lack of preparation by the hospital and insufficient PPE. What's more, the lab samples were sent in the same manner as all other samples, with no additional protections.

Responding to the director's remarks that the nurses broke protocol, Rose Ann DeMoro from the nurse's union stated, "Were protocols breached? There were no protocols."

Pham is now suing Texas Health Presbyterian Hospital. She alleges that the hospital did not do enough to prepare. NBC News reported the following:

> "The sum total of the information Nina was provided
> to protect herself before taking on her patient was what
> her manager 'Googled' and printed out from the Internet,"

the lawsuit says. It also alleges that Pham was told that the protective gear she wore while treating Duncan was safe, and that she was at "no risk" of contracting the disease.

The lawsuit—illustrated with an ominous microscope image of the virus on its first page—also says that the hospital used Pham as a "PR tool" in the face of public scrutiny, and lied that her condition was improving when medical reports told a different story.[2]

Meanwhile, back in Sierra Leone, Liberia, and Guinea, Ebola was still raging. Bodies could be found lying both in the streets and in waiting rooms, where the sick never got a chance to be seen by a doctor. Not all those dying in waiting rooms even had Ebola, but needed medical care of some kind and were unable to get it because of the Ebola outbreak taking up all available resources.

Numerous quarantines were tried in both Sierra Leone and Liberia. During this time, residents had their homes searched by officials looking for individuals with symptoms. Such individuals were removed from the homes for treatment. Unfortunately, none of these quarantines could stop the spread of Ebola. They only fostered further anger and mistrust between the people and their governments.

It's difficult to keep people in quarantine for much longer than a few days. Hunger is a strong motivator for people to break quarantine, and these quarantines happened in places of great poverty, like the slum of West Point, Liberia. Violence is common with these quarantines.

In the face of clinic attacks, deadly disease, lack of equipment, and lack of funds to pay staff, health care workers had to make a choice whether to come to work or to stay home. Some stayed home. In Sierra Leone, one hospital's workers went on strike over the lack of supplies and lack of pay.

2   http://www.nbcnews.com/storyline/ebola-virus-outbreak/nina-pham-nurse-who-survived-ebola-sues-texas-hospital-n315776.

US Government and Media Response

During the fall of 2014, the media was awash with Ebola stories and mentions of Ebola by politicians. This crisis happened to coincide with the US midterm elections. Much of the media coverage of the Ebola pandemic seemed to fall neatly along the typical political dividing lines, with media outlets catering to the liberal Left downplaying the risks of Ebola and attempting to make the issue about conservatives who didn't like President Barack Obama, as if one had anything to do with the other. Those media outlets catering to the conservative Right presented the Ebola pandemic as a clear and present danger to every household in the United States, and that it was coming to a neighborhood near you next week.

This type of agenda-driven response, regardless of which extreme, is counterproductive. On the one hand, you have people who take the risk far too seriously and who will act out of fear. On the other, you have people who do not take the risk seriously enough and will function based on normalcy bias. Neither is a rational approach.

Toward the end of October, President Obama announced his appointment of Ron Klain, a Fannie Mae lobbyist known for his ability to circumnavigate the bureaucracy of Washington, DC, and government regulations, as Ebola response coordinator, a position often referred to in the media as the "Ebola czar."

Within a matter of weeks, the United States got an Ebola czar, the midterm elections were held, and Ebola was out of the news. The Associated Press released a statement that was sent to editors on how it would handle reporting on Ebola. There were to be no more stories on suspected Ebola unless that suspected case caused some major upset or delay. Suddenly, all stories of suspected cases of Ebola were gone from mainstream news coverage.

The Future of Ebola

The last anyone heard about Ebola, unless you've been actively digging for the information, was that the United States was sending in our military to provide the supplies, labor, and training necessary to combat the spread of Ebola in West Africa. That was all. The media moved on, and most people in the United States forgot about Ebola. What had been a major story for months was quickly and quietly gone. Unfortunately, the Ebola pandemic itself has gone nowhere, and people are still dying in Guinea, Sierra Leone, and Liberia.

It has been over a year since the first case of Ebola was reported in Guinea. Since then, Ebola has crossed international borders, thereby qualifying it as a pandemic. And while Ebola did make its way to other nations, like Mali and Nigeria, the response there was swift and the outbreaks quickly contained. Recently, WHO has come under heavy criticism for its lack of swift and adequate response at the very beginning of the outbreak.

According to CDC, in the three countries most affected by the current pandemic, there have been over 26,298 cases of Ebola, with 10,892 deaths as of May 1, 2015. There is still no cure. There was the promise implied with experimental drugs, like ZMapp, and there was always the promise of a vaccine that was perpetually "being developed." The vaccine always seemed just around the corner, but has yet to materialize over a year later. Researchers may finally be close to getting a vaccine approved. WHO announced that the vaccine was testing well so far. Let's hope that will translate into a fast track for vaccine approval. But for ZMapp, there's still no evidence on whether it's safe and effective. How can it be possible, with tens of thousands of people sick and dying from Ebola in Guinea, Liberia, and Sierra Leone to this day, that there has not been an opportunity to thoroughly test ZMapp? Perhaps there was just more interest in producing a vaccine.

The numbers in Guinea, Sierra Leone, and Liberia are still rising. When an area is cleared of Ebola, within weeks new cases pop up again. This isn't just the longest Ebola outbreak in history anymore. If this situation doesn't change soon, Ebola may become as endemic to this region as cholera and malaria already are. The population, already living in poverty and slums, may well collapse. This would leave a vacuum of control over the region's mining industries. Some of the mines are already being seized or bought out, such as the iron ore mines in Sierra Leone. There are also gold and diamond mines in the region vulnerable to seizure. But will anyone want to work the mines at Ebola's ground zero?

In May 2015, *The Dallas Morning News* released a report that got precious little public attention. There had been an additional twelve people hospitalized in Dallas, nine of them hospital workers, than had been reported. The official reason for this was to protect patient confidentiality. The twelve individuals were reported to all have symptoms matching Ebola, but tested negative. Several individuals had returned to the United States from West Africa and required treatment but were able to remain anonymous even though the media reported that a new case was being treated here. There were also frequent reports of anonymous cases all over the United States and Canada of people who had come from West Africa exhibiting symptoms of Ebola and were very quickly reported as testing negative for Ebola.

This all happened to coincide with Klain's appointment. It's fair to speculate that this had less to do with a desire to protect patient privacy and more to do with the implementation of Klain's apparent management strategy: silence.

What Can We Learn From the Ebola Pandemic?

A number of important points stand out.

- Local and global response to a potential pandemic may be slow and inadequate.
- Official response may be more about keeping people calm and not about keeping people safe.
- Our local hospitals are likely to be unprepared for a deadly infectious disease.

- Local hospitals are likely to be lacking in an established and practiced protocol for this level of threat.
- When hospitals reach capacity, everyone's health is at risk because of dwindling resources.
- When people are afraid, they can become violent and prone to believing the worst.
- Everything has a political angle.
- Everything has a monetary angle.
- If there are experimental drugs, they will be reserved for only certain individuals.
- When things get out of hand, expect martial law in the form of curfews, quarantines, and door-to-door searches.
- When people are hungry, they can become violent and dangerous.
- Areas with a high population density are more risky.
- Officials are more concerned with assigning blame than assuming responsibility.
- Pandemic threats exist, even if the media isn't reporting them.
- If a situation seems too horrible and too awful, many people will fall back to normalcy bias and just refuse to acknowledge what's happening right in front of them.
- You will need a plan of your own for survival.

If the tragedy of this Ebola pandemic has taught us anything, it's that we must prepare. Our government has a history of slow and inadequate response to natural and human-made disasters. Why should a pandemic, any pandemic, be any different? And keep in mind, while there's a lot to learn from this Ebola outbreak, this isn't just about Ebola. New diseases emerge. Old diseases resurge. Pathogens develop immunity to our drugs. Let this be your wake-up call.

CHAPTER 2

Pandemic Preparation 101:
Overview, Terminology, General Pandemic Concerns

This chapter is intended to provide background on core concepts, such as what pandemics are, how infectious disease is spread, and how the threat of a large-scale, deadly, infectious disease affects our preparedness decisions.

Pandemics have happened throughout history. There are pandemics happening right now. There will be pandemics in the future. They do not necessarily follow any pattern and can happen without warning. All it takes is for just the right mutation to take place, and we have a pandemic on our hands. Pandemics happen, so what do you need to know about them?

Pandemic versus Epidemic

The internationally accepted definition of a pandemic is "an epidemic occurring worldwide, or over a very wide area, crossing international boundaries and usually affecting a large number of people."[3] WHO also has set the following three criteria for a pandemic:

- Able to infect humans.
- Able to cause disease in humans.
- Able to spread from human to human quite easily.

A pandemic, then, is determined by how far and how easily an epidemic disease is spread in humans, not by its severity. Pandemics are epidemics that infect a larger region. An epidemic is an infectious disease that has crossed borders. This doesn't always mean thousands of miles, especially in the case of smaller countries. With the United States, one can go thousands of miles without crossing borders. The distinction between *pandemic* and *epidemic* becomes blurred.

For example, if an outbreak of influenza were to run rampant in Pennsylvania, infecting a high concentration of individuals in Pennsylvania, this would be an epidemic. But if it were to spread across the country or spill over into Mexico or Canada, or travel by plane to parts unknown, and the disease then spreads in the new country, this has transitioned from an epidemic to a pandemic. In common usage, the terms *pandemic* and *epidemic* are more fluid and flexible. Again, severity of the illness is not a factor in whether a disease is considered a pandemic disease.

Current Threats

When it comes to current threats, we already have multiple diseases that qualify as active pandemics, whether or not CDC or WHO has acknowledged them all. Some of these include Ebola, HIV/AIDS, tuberculosis, and viral hepatitis.

There are also numerous, current epidemics all over the planet that could spread and transition into the classification of pandemic. There are seasonal epidemics, such as influenza, that eventually work their way around the globe. There are diseases that WHO is monitoring, such

---

3   *Dictionary of Epidemiology*, 4th ed. (Oxford University Press, 2001).

as cholera, malaria, meningitis, yellow fever, plague, and coronaviruses (like SARS and MERS).

New Threats

New threats are constantly emerging, and old threats are resurging. The major culprits here are emerging diseases, zoonotic diseases, and antibiotic-resistant "superbugs."

Emerging Diseases

We just don't know much about any emerging diseases. By the time we learn what's causing the illness and how it's transmitted, the outbreak could have already spread widely. Powassan, which is spread by ticks, is one to keep an eye on. Considering how widespread and prevalent ticks are, Powassan has the potential to become an epidemic and ultimately a pandemic.

Zoonotic Diseases

These are diseases that pass from animals to humans, such as avian flu (H5N1, H7N9), which comes from infected birds, and swine flu (H1N1). Middle East respiratory syndrome (MERS), which is a coronavirus that initially spread to humans from camels and then mutated to spread from person to person. Ebola virus is thought, though not proved, to be spread by eating undercooked "bushmeat," such as monkeys or bats.

Drug-Resistant Bacteria

CDC is monitoring multiple bacterial diseases that have demonstrated an ability to resist antibiotic drug therapy, also known as "superbugs." These are varying degrees of resistance, including drug-resistant (DR), multidrug-resistant (MDR), extensively drug-resistant (XDR), and totally drug-resistant (TDR).

Drug-resistant bacteria will get a more thorough treatment later in this book. But it's important to note here that certain bacteria that were once easy to treat, such as those that cause gonorrhea, are now presenting a challenge. In fact, CDC has listed drug-resistant *Neisseria gonorrhoeae*, the bacteria that causes gonorrhea, as an "urgent threat."[4] Considering how easily this bacteria is transmitted, there's good reason to take every precaution to prevent getting gonorrhea in the first place.

Because the United States doesn't see nearly the number of tuberculosis cases seen in other parts of the world, it's tempting to think that it's a defeated disease. However, CDC's 2013 threat report lists drug-resistant *Mycobacterium tuberculosis*, the bacteria responsible for causing tuberculosis (TB), as a "serious threat," and this report doesn't even include the MDR TB, XDR TB, or worse still, TDR TB found in places like India, which just happens to also have the second-largest population in the world.

We also see regular staph infections of methicillin-resistant *Staphylococcus aureus* (MRSA) in people who receive treatment in hospitals for other illnesses. Health care–acquired MRSA is the most common source of MRSA in the United States. However, community-acquired MRSA is also happening more frequently. MDR *Escherichia coli* and MDR salmonella (both nontyphoidal and typhoidal) present significant danger.

The Next Great Pandemic

Deadly disease and disaster go hand in hand. Where there's one, you'll find the other. Many diseases we no longer worry about because of our modern infrastructure and medical system. But without such support, these diseases would reappear in a hurry. There are also diseases that are evolving and adapting, and seem poised to break out all over the globe irrespective of our advances. In this section, I examine diseases that follow disaster, as well as diseases with the potential to be the disaster. Starting with the latter, let's take a look at what may be the next great pandemic.

---

4   http://www.cdc.gov/drugresistance/pdf/ar-threats-2013-508.pdf.

My Top Picks for the Next Great Pandemic

The following list of infectious diseases is based on current outbreaks, current threats, and historical information. There are two primary categories: drug-resistant bacteria and viruses known to mutate easily and frequently. Some of these are zoonotic infections, which are transmitted to humans from an animal or insect.

I also took into account potential pandemic diseases that could be unleashed into the human population either on purpose, as in the case of terrorism, or by accident, such as by human error permitting a deadly illness to escape from a laboratory.

My list for the most likely candidates for the next great pandemic include:

- Influenza
- Tuberculosis
- Methicillin-resistant *Staphylococcus aureus*, aka MRSA
- Coronaviruses (SARS, MERS)
- Viral hemorrhagic fever (Ebola, Marburg, Lassa)
- Diseases spread by terrorism/human error (smallpox, plague)
- The Surprise

In the chapters that follow, I have provided an outline of each disease, explaining why it made the list. There's also a symptoms and transmission section to help recognize the illness and, I hope, prevent its spread. Finally, there's a response section with suggestions on how to prepare yourself and your family/group for such an eventuality.

In this chapter, as well as in the next, we see both bacterial and viral infections. To understand these better, let's take a moment to discuss what these microorganisms are and how they spread.

BACTERIA

Bacteria are microorganisms, too tiny to see with the naked eye. They're one of the oldest forms of life on earth and have adapted to just about every environment, no matter how inhospitable. Bacteria are literally everywhere, in the soil, water, air, and even radioactive waste. Bacteria live on you and inside you. And most of the time, this is exactly how it should be. Sometimes, however, when a type of bacteria becomes dominant in a landscape, or in a body, we see illness.

Bacteria have symbiotic and parasitic relationships with their hosts. In the case of healthy or "friendly" bacteria, they can keep us healthy. Healthy gut bacteria are necessary for proper digestion and feed on things such as other bacteria and yeasts, like candida. Symbiotic bacteria help keep candida populations in check. Bacteria in lacto-fermented foods, such as yogurt, sauerkraut, and kefir, help keep our gut bacteria balanced and our intestines functioning well.

Other bacteria, such as *Mycobacterium tuberculosis*, which causes the disease called tuberculosis, can be deadly. In this case, the body is providing the medium in which the bacteria are allowed to grow and spread while the person deteriorates. This is a parasitic relationship where only one side, the bacteria, is benefiting from the relationship.

Bacteria are single-cell organisms that replicate quickly. The cell grows and then divides fast enough to double its numbers every twenty minutes. This single cell is covered by a cell membrane, which holds in things the bacteria needs, such as nutrients. The cell membrane is covered by a cell wall. The cell membrane and cell wall form the cell envelope. It's this envelope that antibiotic drugs must penetrate to gain access to the bacteria's cell to kill it, if possible.

There are gram-positive and gram-negative bacteria. Hans Christian Gram was a bacteriologist who developed a method of staining bacteria, which then categorized bacteria as either positive or negative. The difference between the two has mostly to do with the type of cell wall the bacteria has, whether it's thicker and smooth or thin and wavy. Antibiotic drugs tend to be effective for one category of bacteria or the other, which is important to know for proper treatment.

The Threat of Antibiotic Resistance

What we are seeing today is that medicines that were once highly effective at killing these bacteria, and which often kill beneficial bacteria as well, are becoming less and less effective. This has happened for several reasons, including overprescription of antibiotics, patients not completing their full course of antibiotics, overuse of antibiotic disinfectants, disposal of medications into the water supply, improper use of antibiotics in agriculture, and lack of newer-generation antibiotics.

Overprescription of Antibiotics. I recall when I was a young girl having to go to the doctor for a sore throat. I was expecting that awful swab test for strep throat when the doctor told my mother, "I'm just going to write a prescription for antibiotics. If she has strep throat, then it's better for her to get the antibiotics right away. If it's not, then no worries. It's not like taking these are going to do any harm."

For decades in the United States and elsewhere in the developed world where antibiotic medications have been available, this was the policy. Prescribe the antibiotic just in case. But we now know that there were unintended consequences of that advice. Taking unnecessary antibiotic medications can weaken the immune system by disrupting our internal flora. But it also means that we expose bacteria in our environment to doses of antibiotic drugs far more frequently than necessary. This speeds up the rate at which bacteria adapt.

The thing about bacteria is that they're smart. They've demonstrated the abilities to communicate and cooperate, and with different types of bacteria, not just their own strain or even their own species. Bacteria have several mechanisms by which they communicate with other bacteria they encounter, one of which being bacteria-infecting viruses. When a virus infects bacteria, it learns its defense mechanisms. This information is then transmitted through the viral replication and encounters with other bacteria.

Every encounter between bacteria and an antibiotic drug increases the bacteria's ability to resist that drug in the future. Every encounter, even when antibiotics are used appropriately.

Failure to Finish Entire Course of Antibiotics. When a sick person does have a bacterial infection, antibiotics are appropriate. But it's imperative that the patient complete the entire course of antibiotics. It's tempting to stop taking the antibiotic pills once a patient starts to feel better. When this happens, some of the bacteria survive, mutate, and infect another person. In fact, only the strongest of bacteria remain to replicate. When the bacteria infect another person, it's these stronger bacteria that infect the new patient. The process is then repeated and repeated until the antibiotic drug no longer has any effect on the bacteria.

Overuse of Antibacterial Soaps, Hand Sanitizers, and Disinfectants. In addition to coming in contact with antibiotic drugs in treating a sick patient, bacteria have been assaulted with a barrage of antibacterial agents. Bacteria have been able to share information about these agents and develop resistance. This resistance turns places such as hospitals, which use the most thorough disinfectants to protect their patients, into factories for some of the most resistant bacteria.

Soap is not always antibacterial, and it doesn't have to be. Soap cleans through the creation of friction. The friction physically removes microorganisms. Hand washing needs to be done properly, but it's a more sustainable way to keep pathogenic microorganisms off our hands and bodies.

Hand sanitizers can be a great option for when there's no water. But what has happened in hospitals is that hand sanitizers have become a quick way to get around proper hand washing. Instead of killing all the bacteria on hospital staff's hands, it ends up being applied in haste, in insufficient amounts, and the bacteria get a low dose to which they adapt.

Antibiotics in the Water Supply. Antibiotics, along with many other medications, are routinely disposed of down toilets. This may happen when a patient is prescribed a new medication and the antibiotic is no longer being taken. The remaining medications are then disposed of in hospitals, nursing homes, group homes, and other care facilities by flushing them down the toilet.

These antibiotics enter the water supply and create a perpetual low dose of antibiotic medicating for all who drink it and any bacteria that come in contact with that municipal water supply. The constant exposure to low-dose antibiotics creates the perfect storm for antibiotic resistance to develop. Every exposure matters.

Antibiotics in the Food Supply. Outside the hospital setting, the number one source of antibiotic resistance comes from factory farms and their practices that take place in confined animal feeding operations (CAFOs). According to a January 2001 article from *Scientific American*,

"Most US Antibiotics Fed to Healthy Livestock,"[5] over 70 percent of all antibiotics in the United States are used in modern agriculture's meat production. Nothing has been done to stop the practice, even fourteen years later. In fact, it has only worsened. In 2013 the percentage was up to 80 percent.[6]

The use of antibiotics in livestock is intended to help spur faster-than-normal growth, thereby increasing profit. Low-dose antibiotics in the feed result in bigger, fatter animals faster. But that has produced drug-resistant *Escherichia coli* (E. coli), *Salmonella typhi*, and nontyphoid salmonella. These superbugs have found their way into waterways, the meat during butchering, the food packaging plants, and ultimately, onto our plates.

Lack of Newer-Generation Antibiotics. To make matters worse, the pharmaceutical industry has neglected research and development of newer generations of antibiotics. From an industry viewpoint, antibiotics are used for short periods of time, usually ten to fourteen days, sometimes longer for illnesses like Lyme disease or tuberculosis. But why would they do this when they could invest those same research and development resources into the next maintenance drug? The money is in maintenance drugs, not antibiotics. So instead of a drug for a single course of strep throat, research goes into the next diabetes, high blood pressure, cholesterol, or antidepressant drug that people will take daily for presumably the rest of their lives. This is an extremely shortsighted viewpoint, and one that will come back to bite us.

Bacteria are smart. Frighteningly smart. These single-cell microorganisms adapt and communicate what they've learned to other bacteria, resulting in the ever-growing list of diseases thought to be defeated and now reemerging. They share information as easily as we communicate online through e-mail and social media.

Antibiotic resistance can take several forms. Sometimes, the bacteria have developed a way to screen out the drug that might attach to something the bacteria would normally permit to pass through the

5   http://www.scientificamerican.com/article/most-us-antibiotics-fed-t.
6   http://archinte.jamanetwork.com/article.aspx?articleid=1738717.

cell envelope and beyond the cell membrane. Other times, the bacteria have developed a way to degrade the drug and render it useless. Some bacteria have developed a type of pump, a multidrug resistant efflux pump (MDR efflux pump), that pushes the antibiotic out of the cell. Finally, and most disturbingly, some bacteria have developed a way to alter the target of the antibiotic. The antibiotic is allowed into the cell, where it does absolutely nothing.

At this point, I would suggest that anyone who's serious about being prepared for a pandemic should not only stock up on antibiotics, usually obtained as fish antibiotics, but also study herbal medicine. There are many effective options for alternatives to antibiotics in the world of botanical and natural medicine. Plants have also had to adapt and evolve alongside bacteria and bacterial threats. This is something that a pharmaceutical drug cannot claim. Once a drug is formulated, that's is. It doesn't change. This makes it easier for the bacteria to develop resistance. With a good supply of both conventional antibiotics and herbal antibiotics, you'll be well equipped to face a bacterial threat.

The other major threat presented by antibiotic resistance is that without effective antibiotics, many of our medical advances are gone. Modern surgery as we know it—over. Organ transplants? No more. Surgery, even lifesaving, necessary or you-will-die surgery, would leave you vulnerable to infections, especially virulent and vigorous bacteria that have evolved over the past century.

There's no way around it. Antibiotic resistance is a major threat. It may well be TDR TB, MRSA, or even typhoid that takes us out. That is, if a virus doesn't do it first.

VIRUSES

Viruses are even smaller than bacteria. They're the absolute bare bones of what it takes to be considered "alive," although to be fair, there are those who don't consider viruses alive.

Where bacteria are a single-cell organism, a virus is a single strand of DNA or RNA, sometimes covered in a protective envelope of protein. DNA viruses replicate in very stable ways. It is the RNA viruses, however, that do not. They mutate more easily and more quickly. The envelope of protein surrounding some viruses acts as a protective layer, almost like a seed's coat.

If we stay with the seed analogy, once in the body, the virus must plant itself. It penetrates human cells, just like a seed penetrates the soil. Once planted in our cells, the virus can replicate and send itself into other cells, like a network of roots.

The virus then takes snippets of either DNA or RNA, as well as leaving behind DNA and RNA. It forms a type of web connecting each of us to each other. It's quite a fascinating process. Unfortunately, sometimes this leaves us very sick.

Developing antiviral medication is challenging. How do you develop medicine that can seek out and destroy a harmful virus embedded in living cells without also damaging those cells? Most standard treatments of viral respiratory infections rely on at-home care, with the standard advice of get plenty of rest, drink lots of fluids, take a decongestant, take a pain reliever/fever reducer (which isn't always good advice) to minimize the symptoms, and seek treatment again if there's no relief within a week.

If symptoms persist, then oxygen and IV fluids are usually given at a hospital. If any antiviral medications were appropriate, they would be given. But for the most part, the hospital is only going to administer oxygen, monitor vital signs, and do what it can to keep air passages clear. The patient has to fight the infection off on his or her own.

The primary way our modern medical system has chosen to approach viruses is by vaccination. Though some vaccines are intended to fight bacterial infections, vaccines have been developed for a range of viruses; most familiar to us are those for childhood diseases like measles and the mumps.

Some of these vaccines are truly lifesaving. I don't think anyone would deny the benefit of getting a tetanus shot versus getting tetanus, or the benefit of having a rabies shot available right after a bite from a potentially rabid animal. Others, such as the chicken pox vaccine or the HPV vaccine, may be doing more harm than good. But vaccines are not a 100 percent slam-dunk solution. Viruses that mutate frequently are notoriously difficult to develop an effective vaccine for. Vaccines also take time, measured in months, not weeks, before a viable formula can be developed. And again, there's the economic factor: pharmaceutical companies have little incentive to create vaccines for many diseases, especially those diseases that affect the poorest of populations. There just isn't much money to be made selling a malaria vaccine to people who have no money to pay for it.

As with my suggestion above for preparedness against bacterial infections, I would strongly recommend studying herbal medicine. There are herbs that are highly antiviral and may help people survive a deadly viral outbreak.

Please note: in this book, I refer to people who are sick as patients. Unless you're a licensed physician, you cannot call anyone your patient. In a disaster, however, such distinctions between licensed providers and other knowledgeable people will be blurred in the interests of helping the sick. For the unique circumstances discussed in this book, the term *patient* seems more appropriate and less cumbersome than "the sick person."

How Does Disease Spread?

The spread of any disease happens with a pathogenic microorganism, either a bacteria, a virus, a fungus, or a parasite, that moves into healthy people and makes them unwell. This generally happens through one of the following kinds of contact.

Direct Contact

Person to Person. This type of contact includes airborne transmission (influenza in the tiny water droplets that remain in the air after a cough), exchange of bodily fluids (tuberculosis in the saliva while sharing a piece of pizza), sexual intercourse (HIV/AIDS), and blood transfusions or contact with blood (hepatitis).

Animal/Insect to Person. This type of transmission can be from either your pet or a wild animal, or perhaps an insect. Examples of these are rabies, often found in bats, raccoons, feral cats, and dogs. Anytime you see an animal acting peculiarly, avoid it. The dying animal has an overwhelming urge to bite to pass on the virus. Insect bites can bring Lyme disease, Powassan, West Nile virus, malaria, and eastern equine encephalitis (EEE).

Rodents are well known for spreading disease. They can carry fleas that in turn infect humans with bubonic plague, which is something that's more prevalent in the western United States. Rodents can be infected with hantavirus, leptospirosis, Lassa, tularemia, plus a variety of hemorrhagic fevers, and spread it to humans through their urine and feces. Most of the time, their urine or feces contaminate food or water. But hantavirus and the various hemorrhagic fevers are contracted by inhaling dust contaminated by urine or feces.

Vertical Transmission (Mother to Unborn Child or during Birth). Several illnesses can cross the placenta and infect the child prior to birth or during birth. In addition to whatever risks the mother may face from the illness, there's also a risk to the developing child. There could be congenital defects, such as hearing loss, more severe birth defects, or worse, the loss of the pregnancy.

One way to remember some of these diseases that can cross the placenta is the acronym "CHEAPTORCHES," which stands for:

- Chicken pox (and shingles)
- Hepatitis (all types but A)
- Enteroviruses (polio)
- AIDS/HIV
- Parvovirus
- Toxoplasmosis
- Other (Coxsackievirus, Lyme disease, listeria, group B strep)
- Rubella
- Cytomegalovirus
- Herpes simplex
- Everything else sexually transmitted
- Syphilis

Indirect Contact

This type of contact involves at least one step between the carrier and the infected person. This is often a doorknob or other surface where a sick person or animal has left the infectious microorganism. For instance, a person coughs into his or her hand and touches a door handle, elevator button, furniture, or some other surface. Another person comes along, touches the same surface, and then touches his or her face. The infection is either inhaled or perhaps migrates to the mucous membranes of the mouth, nose, or eyes.

Sometimes, the indirect contact is through an animal. Rodents are also part of how tick-borne and mosquito-borne illnesses spread. Infected ticks bite the rodents, and tick larvae attach themselves to mice, chipmunks, and other small animals. When the larvae feed on an infected mouse, they become infected, and the cycle continues. The larger the rodent population, the larger the infected tick population.[7] The same can be said for West Nile virus.

Note: Rodent control is an essential part of minimizing risk during a pandemic or severe epidemic.

Food/Water Contamination

Food and water can become contaminated and easily lead to illness. E. coli, salmonella, certain strains of listeria, giardia, cholera, cryptosporidiosis, and shigella are just some of the food-borne and waterborne illnesses we can get from contaminated food and water. These infections produce diarrhea and intestinal cramping, and will raise the risk of serious dehydration. Dehydration could prove fatal depending on circumstances.

---

7   http://journals.plos.org/plosbiology/article?id=10.1371/journal.pbio.0040182.

How to Prevent the Spread of Disease

We may not always know exactly what the disease might be. For example, in a postdisaster situation, or in a remote area with no access to a laboratory for testing, many of the waterborne illnesses will look the same. It'll be equally challenging to distinguish one respiratory infection from another because they'll share many of the same symptoms.

But knowing how diseases spread gives us plenty of clues on how to avoid getting sick, even when we're not sure what the illness is. At least, most of the time. The better you and your community are at preventing, recognizing, and responding to an epidemic or a pandemic outbreak, the better for everyone. These methods include isolation, cleanliness, and waste disposal.

Isolation

This may mean sheltering in place, or it may mean "bugging out" (leaving an area and heading for a predetermined safe place) to a more remote location. Until you know that an illness is not airborne, you must act as if it were. Until you know what the incubation period is for an illness, you must assume even well people may be infected and contagious. If you have symptoms, cover your mouth and nose when you cough and sneeze. If people around you are coughing and sneezing, have some kind of scarf, handkerchief, or even a respiratory mask with which to cover your nose and mouth.

Depending on the outbreak's severity, you may want to evacuate. During the plagues of the medieval period, European nobility and royalty would leave the cities to "vacation" at their country homes, thereby avoiding the plague, which was rampant in the crammed streets and homes of the cities. If the outbreak is serious and deadly enough, it may be wise to retreat to a less-populated area. Population density matters during a pandemic.

If you do choose to retreat to your country cottage, cabin in the woods, and so forth, you'll need to have a plan in place ahead of time for how you'll deal with people who show up after you arrive at your base camp. The group you arrived with, presumably your immediate family, will be healthy. But you can't be sure of anyone who arrives after you.

There are many approaches you can take. You can turn everyone away. You can welcome them with open arms. Those you turn away could come back to haunt you. Those whom you welcome and provide a care package for before they set out again could also come back to haunt you. Expect people to be upset no matter how you react.

If family or friends are supposed to meet you at your base camp, then you need to have a system of quarantine in place before they can fully join your group. I would suggest three to four weeks in a separate camp area. That should be sufficient for most known illnesses to start showing symptoms, including something as exotic and deadly as Ebola. It should cover you for most cases of tuberculosis as well, but tuberculosis can remain latent for weeks, months, even years before developing into active TB. Most cases will become apparent in a matter of weeks.

Another aspect of avoiding contact is to make sure that everyone has their own towels, soap, bed linens, and so on. The last thing you want is to be accidentally cross-contaminating your children's beds or towels. Consider how close to their noses and mouths these linens get. Having their own linens and hygiene supplies helps provide another degree of separation, even when you're living under the same roof.

Finally, make sure that you have proper ventilation. Recirculating air that may be carrying an aerosoled virus through your home or work space is not a good idea. A virus is "aerosoled" when it is dispersed into the air on the small water droplets that escape when a sick person sneezes or coughs. This can often be the fear with a weaponized virus and terrorism. If you can't avoid such a situation, face masks may be helpful.

Cleanliness

Most illnesses can be avoided simply by maintaining high standards for cleanliness. Thankfully, you can clean and disinfect most pathogens simply and with just soap and bleach.

Soap is your number one weapon in the fight against most pathogens. And when I say soap, I mean regular soap, not antibacterial soap. Antibacterial soap and hand-sanitizing gels are contributing to antibiotic resistance. Avoid them. Regular, plain soap cleans by creating friction. This friction lifts dirt, grease, and microorganisms from the skin, which are then rinsed off with water. Instead of attempting to kill the bacteria and viruses on your hands, clothing, or some surface, the friction from the soap removes the pathogen. Hand washing will significantly cut down on the spread of germs. Consider how frequently we touch our faces. Every time we do, we risk transferring germs on our fingertips and hands to our nose, mouth, or eyes. It can be almost impossible to stop touching our faces. Frequent hand washing mitigates the risk of spreading germs by removing germs through friction.

Proper hand-washing technique includes the following:

- Wet hands with water, preferably clean, running water, either warm or cold.
- Rub hands to build lather. This creates friction. Make sure to lather the backs of hands and in between fingers. Work the lather under your nails.
- Continue to wash (lather) hands for twenty seconds.
- Rinses hands off in clean, running water.
- Dry hands, either by air-drying or with a towel.

If there's one skill I recommend all preppers learn, it's how to make soap. It's easy to stock up on a lot of soap, but you don't know what emergencies are coming down the road, how long they'll last, or whether you can guarantee that your supplies will remain secure. Even primitive soap, made with leftover, home-rendered fats and homemade lye from wood ash, is worth knowing how to make. The ability to clean yourself, clothing, linens, and surroundings is vital to preventing the spread of disease.

To help reduce the spread of respiratory illness, if children have already become sick, teach them to sneeze or cough into their elbow instead of their hand to cut down on the spread of germs. This way, their hands will stay cleaner and less likely to leave germs behind on surfaces. Make sure to dispose of all tissues promptly.

Where soap removes germs, bleach kills them. Using soap and then following up with bleach will solve most contamination issues. Other options you could employ include sunlight (for waterborne pathogens), heat (fire or boiling water), and alcohol (wiping down surfaces, dehydrating body fluids on surfaces).

Vinegar, alcohol, and essential oils can kill many microorganisms, but none of these are as effective as bleach. What they do have over bleach is their storage abilities, as chlorine must be used within six months of purchase. If you need to use natural ingredients for your disinfectant, I would use a 5 percent dilution of thyme essential oil in a 50/50 mix of vinegar and sterile water. This oil is an irritant, so keep it away from the skin at this strength. Other options might include oregano oil, peppermint oil, or even a very strong brew of these herbs if you have no other way to clean your environment. But even essential oils and herbs begin to lose their effectiveness after one year.

An easy, affordable solution to the short shelf life of liquid bleach is to make your chlorine bleach at home from a commonly found product called "pool shock." Chlorine bleach that you buy at the store is actually a highly diluted product of mostly water and a tiny bit of sodium hypochlorite. The sodium hypochlorite is actually only 3 percent to 6 percent of the total volume. Pool shock is calcium hypochlorite.

A US Army technical bulletin, "Sanitary Control and Surveillance of Field Water Supplies" (TB MED 577), explains how to make homemade bleach with calcium hypochlorite for disinfecting surfaces and fabrics. You'll need calcium hypochlorite with at least 70 percent available chlorine. You can find pool shock easily with 73 percent available chlorine. Mix 2 level tablespoons of calcium hypochlorite in 3 cups of water to reach a concentration similar to that of store-bought liquid bleach. When using this or any bleach solution, be sure to allow thirty minutes before wiping down the surface for full effect.

Once you've made your own chlorine bleach, you can use and store it exactly as you would for regular, store-bought bleach. It'll have a shelf life of about six months when stored between 50°F and 70°F. You can store this in a bottle that once held chlorine bleach or in some other bottle that can handle corrosive materials.

To disinfect water for drinking, use 8 drops of bleach to 1 gallon of water. Let it set for thirty minutes. I found a great tip on the Survival Mom blog to duct tape an eyedropper to your bleach bottle and use a sharpie to write on the bottle "To Disinfect Water for Drinking: Add 8 drops of bleach per 1 gallon of water." This way, there's no risk of using the eyedropper for something else, and anyone going to use it will know how. I would also write on the bottle when the solution was mixed.

If the water is cloudy, try filtering it through a cloth like a bandanna or T-shirt, repeat the 8 drops of bleach, and wait another thirty minutes. When the water is clear, it's safe to drink. The chlorine will evaporate out of the water. Just let it sit, preferably with a cloth or T-shirt covering it, to allow the gas out but prevent dust or anything else from getting in, for twenty-four hours. This is a common practice of gardeners and those who keep fish tanks who need to remove chlorine from tap water to maintain soil health and to not poison their fish.

With clean water, soap, and bleach, you can clean everything you need to from your hands to doorknobs and counters, to disinfecting bed linens of a sick person. Since bleach can remove colors from fabrics, and it's easier to spot stains on white, try to stock up on white bed linens and towels if you have the choice.

Disposal of Waste

Waste disposal during a pandemic is both vital and problematic. You must be able to dispose of human excrement and daily trash safely. Human waste can be anything from a used tissue from someone with the flu, to a portable toilet for someone with explosive diarrhea, to the remains of those who do not survive. The fluids, remains, or both of a sick person must be dealt with in a manner that prevents spreading the illness to anyone else.

But waste removal services, like curbside trash pickup, can be disrupted during a crisis. Public utilities, such as water, can be shut down if not enough employees are willing or able to go to work. Without water, you're not going to be able to flush your toilet. If you're dependent on public services such as a water utility or curbside trash pickup, you'll need a backup plan for disposing of your waste.

Many rural people are on a septic system. While these work quite well, be mindful that septic systems can back up and that septic maintenance services may not be available during a pandemic. While times are good, make sure that it's well maintained. That way you have at least a couple of years before you might need it pumped. Otherwise, if it backs up into your home, you'll have a major problem on your hands.

There are other options for human waste, some of which are ideal for those living far off the beaten path. There are incinerating toilets and composting toilets on the market that negate the need for a septic system. You can also build your own composting toilet system. An incinerating toilet would be ideal if there are sick people at your location, as it would reduce the waste to ash. But they do require electricity. If you opt for a composting toilet, someone will have to deal with emptying the waste. Outhouses are still in use in many rural areas of the United States and are a solid, low-tech, low-cost option for dealing with human waste.

Some general guidelines for handling such waste with an outhouse or anaerobic composting toilet include the following:

- Use lime, sawdust, or cedar shavings to reduce moisture and odor. Odor will attract flies, which can spread microorganisms from the waste to wherever they land.
- Empty the waste into a hole. Dig the waste hole at least 4 feet deep, but no deeper than chest high for the person digging the hole. If the sides cave in during building, this will prevent the digger from being buried alive.
- Make sure to dig your hole at least 200 feet from any water source or encampment.
- Dig your hole downwind of living quarters.
- Do not pour bleach or any chlorine product down the hole. Chlorine and ammonia make for noxious gases.
- Always wear protective clothing and wash hands well after tending to human waste.

The only systems I know of that can guarantee the destruction of pathogens from human waste are those that use sufficient heat to kill the microorganisms. These include an incinerating toilet or a thermophilic composting system for human waste, as described in the book *The Humanure Handbook*, by Joseph Jenkins.

The incinerating toilet turns waste to ash. The thermophilic composting system produces heat sufficient to kill all manner of excreted pathogens, such as E. coli, enteric viruses, worms, cholera vibrio, shigella, and many more.

Food waste is divided into animal food waste and nonanimal food waste. Nonanimal food waste can be added to the compost heap. Animal food waste, such as bones, fat, meat, or dairy, must be handled similarly to human waste. Either it's buried or burned to ash. The only exception to this is eggshell, which can be composted with your nonmeat waste.

Daily trash may include paper, plastics, and any number of broken, opened, and used leftover material. Expect that weekly trash collection and any community-recycling program will cease during a pandemic. Start thinking now about what materials you'll be generating and how they can either be repurposed or disposed of.

For example, papers can be made into paper pulp bricks. While I wouldn't cook with them, they make a good starter for a wood stove. Plastic buckets have tons of uses. They come in various sizes and can be used as washbasins, pots for plants, or a spare composting toilet. Do not burn plastics, Styrofoam, or anything that will give off toxic fumes.

Should You Go to a Hospital during a Pandemic?

As the West African Ebola pandemic showed, medical facilities face incredible challenges during a pandemic. Hospital beds and supplies can be used up faster than they can be replaced. A hospital's ability to handle a sudden influx of patients is known as surge capacity.

In the United States, most hospitals' backup plans for surge capacity involve relocating patients to other hospitals. This isn't going to help in an epidemic or pandemic, as every hospital will be facing the same sudden influx of patients.

As vital as adequate supplies are to caring for the sick, the people who make the hospital work, including the janitorial staff, the nursing staff, the dietary staff, the administrative staff, the ER doctors, and the lab techs, are vital. If hospital staff fall ill, stop coming to work, or both, the facility and its patients will be in extremely serious trouble.

Looking at the lessons we learned from the Ebola outbreak, hospitals that have reached surge capacity may end up sending people to crowded waiting areas with no hope of actually receiving any care. It doesn't matter why they came for treatment. Whether they were women about to give birth, a father experiencing a heart attack, or someone suspected of having Ebola, it didn't matter. There just weren't enough ER beds to go around for everyone and not enough doctors, nurses, or supplies to treat everyone who came in for care.

Another thing to factor into whether you want to go to the hospital for treatment is if the hospital may be a target for violence. The world witnessed multiple attacks on medical facilities in West Africa because of fear over Ebola. We would like to think that we wouldn't react that way. But fear is a powerful motivator, as is anger when loved ones do not survive, and distrust when leadership is less than transparent.

A pandemic is a crisis, and you can be sure that there will be opportunists who will do everything in their power to capitalize on it. There are also many who will take advantage of that fear for their own reasons, like charlatans selling a "cure," those promoting their own particular brand of religious fanaticism, and politicians bickering and posturing for more influence in the community.

I would never say to anyone not to go to a hospital. If that's where you believe that you'll receive the best quality of care, then absolutely, go to the hospital. But during an outbreak of a contagious, deadly disease, one serious enough for you to consider isolating yourself, the hospital may or may not be able to give you the care you expect.

So you need to learn as much as possible about being prepared medically. If you're capable of handling a child's earache or have the skill to clean a wound and suture it when appropriate, you won't have to go to a hospital where there are potentially far greater risks lurking in the waiting room and emergency exam room than what you would face on your own at home.

Granted, there are some emergencies that really require a hospital and a surgeon and modern medical interventions. But unless you're experiencing something like that, where your life is on the line without medical care, you may be better off at home instead of being exposed to a contagious, deadly, pandemic disease.

Of course, this assumes that life was going along fine until the pandemic outbreak hit, and there's even a hospital or clinic in working order available. If a devastating illness happened after another crisis, however, this may be an entirely moot point. If there had been some prior calamity, such as civil unrest, economic collapse, or an electromagnetic pulse (EMP), you can be sure of two things:

- Hospitals and pharmacies will be targets for both looters and different factions in power struggles.
- After a calamity, there will be disease.

After a disaster, there will be some disease, quite possibly because of inappropriate disposal of human waste. Once cold and flu season rolls around, there will be severe respiratory complaints, like influenza, bronchitis, and pneumonia on top of E. coli, salmonella, cholera, and typhoid. We may also encounter travelers from places much farther away and from foreign countries looking to escape what has befallen their homes and bringing illnesses common to their region with them.

For pandemic preparedness, where the pandemic is the disaster or the pandemic follows a disaster, you may have different considerations on whether seeking hospital care is your best option. Being well stocked in medical supplies for various illnesses and injuries, and well trained on how to respond and use your supplies, will allow you greater flexibility in choosing how to get quality medical care in extreme circumstances.

In addition to stocking up on medical supplies and knowing how to use them, let's take a look at how our existing state of health would affect our chances of survival if a pandemic disease came to the neighborhood tomorrow. I'm specifically referring to preexisting conditions.

Preexisting Conditions

While a few illnesses seem to target the healthy, such as the 1918 influenza pandemic, the so-called Spanish flu, most infectious diseases do not. In general, the healthier you are going into an epidemic or pandemic, the better off you're going to be.

The recent MERS outbreak is a perfect example. While there are still a handful of cases in Saudi Arabia, MERS is a disease we are very lucky has not flared up again. MERS is a coronavirus, like SARS. MERS kills 3 to 4 out of 10 people who become infected. That's a 30 to 40 percent mortality rate. While that's alarming, when the disease first started to spread, it appeared to have closer to a 60 percent mortality rate. So, why the 20 to 30 percent decrease in mortality?

In all likelihood, the mortality rate probably didn't drop. It's more likely that the mild cases went undetected at first. But 30 percent mortality is reminiscent of the Spanish flu, where people died mainly from complications of the flu, such as pneumonia.

The early MERS fatalities reveal something interesting. MERS is a zoonotic disease originating in camels. The first individuals to contract MERS were camel herders who were in close contact with camels and drank camel milk as well as camel urine. It also happened that most of these men also had preexisting, chronic conditions. This raised the risk of death from MERS dramatically.

An early study published in the *Lancet* of MERS victims, including forty-seven individuals and one child with laboratory-confirmed MERS coronavirus, produced the following findings:

- Twenty-eight patients died, a 60 percent fatality rate.
- The fatality rate rose with increasing age.
- Only two of the forty-seven cases were previously healthy.
- Most patients (45 [96 percent]) had underlying comorbid medical disorders.

These break down to:

- diabetes (32 [68 percent])
- hypertension (16 [34 percent])

- chronic cardiac disease (13 [28 percent])
- chronic renal disease (23 [49 percent])[8]

We can clearly see that there's an association between MERS being fatal and the deceased having a preexisting chronic illness. Now consider the instance of chronic illness in the United States. According to CDC, one in two adults in America has a chronic illness, and one in four has multiple chronic illnesses.[9] CDC also reports that 9.3 percent of our population have diabetes,[10] 29 percent have hypertension,[11] 11.3 percent have cardiac disease,[12] and 10 percent have chronic renal disease.[13]

So there's a significant portion of the American population at a higher risk of mortality from an infectious disease, such as MERS, because of the high rate of chronic illness already here.

Part of prepping for a pandemic, therefore, must include some plan to reverse any chronic illness or at least improve your health to the best of your ability. You don't have to be a world-class athlete, but improving your current state of health will improve your odds against an infectious disease moving into your area. You may still get sick. But your odds of surviving that illness are better the healthier you are prior to getting sick.

What does this mean? If you're a type 2 diabetic and you need to adjust your diet and exercise more to manage your blood glucose and get better circulation so you can reduce or even eventually discontinue your medication (under your doctor's supervision, of course), then you do so. If you have hypertension, then you make the necessary adjustments to improve it and reduce your dependence on your medication (again, with your doctor's help). If you have a doctor who refuses to help you in this way, then you find another doctor who's interested in cultivating the healthiest you possible, and not just maintaining your current level of sickness. In that case, he or she isn't doing you any favors.

---

8   http://www.thelancet.com/journals/laninf/article/PIIS1473-3099(13)70204-4/fulltext.
9   http://www.cdc.gov/chronicdisease/overview/#ref2.
10 http://www.cdc.gov/features/diabetesfactsheet.
11 http://www.cdc.gov/bloodpressure/facts.htm.
12 http://www.cdc.gov/nchs/fastats/heart-disease.htm.
13 http://www.cdc.gov/diabetes/pubs/pdf/kidney_factsheet.pdf.

CHAPTER 3

Threat Level I:
Influenza, Tuberculosis, & Staphylococcus Aureas

Introduction to Threat Assessment Points

So, what will that next great pandemic be? There are so many possibilities, some bacterial, some viral, some human-made, some incredibly lethal, some active right now, that it was impossible to tell at a glance which threats had a greater probability of materializing. I had to narrow the choices down, and I needed a way to compare apples to oranges.

I devised a point system to assess the risk of potential pandemic threats. The point scale runs from zero to fifteen, with fifteen being the more imminent and deadly threat. This system weighed various factors, added up the points, and found seven that stood out from all the rest: 1) influenza, 2) tuberculosis, 3) methicillin-resistant *Staphylococcus aureus* (MRSA), 4) coronaviruses (SARS, MERS), 5) viral hemorrhagic fevers (VHFs) or Ebola, Marburg, and Lassa 6) diseases spread by terrorism/human error (smallpox, plague) and 7) The Surprise. These seven threats represent what I consider to be the most likely scenarios for the next great pandemic. If you are concerned about pandemics, these seven potential threats are the ones which deserve your attention and preparedness efforts.

Thankfully, there were no contenders that scored a fifteen. The seven contenders which made the cut for this book were clustered between seven and eleven, with one exception being the final consideration of a new, emerging illness. There were many that only reached 5 points or under on this scale, which I did not discuss in this book. Instead, I focused on the cluster with the highest points, representing the greatest pandemic threats, for efficient pandemic preparation.

Factors considered included prior history, such as did this disease ever have a strain that was or is currently a pandemic? How easily can this disease be spread? Do we have any idea how to treat this disease? How deadly is it? What are the odds if a person becomes sick that they will either live or die? Does this disease have a history of mutation? And if so, how often does it mutate?

To further prioritize these seven contenders, I divided them into "threat levels." Threat Level I are those diseases that scored the highest and therefore are of the most concern. Threat Level II scored in the middle, and Threat Level III scored the least. Please remember, all threat levels are to be taken seriously. Remember, there were only a few points difference from the highest threat level to the lowest threat level of these seven potential pandemic candidates.

The Threat Assessment Point Scale can be used with any disease that concerns you. If I haven't covered the illness you are most anxious about, just plug it into the point system to see how it ranks alongside my choices.

A breakdown of the point system I used is as follows.

THREAT ASSESSMENT POINTS		
THREAT	**POINTS**	**DETAILS**
Past Pandemic	1	The disease has caused a pandemic at least once historically.
Current Epidemic	2	The disease is currently active within a specific region, and is highly contagious and deadly.
Current Pandemic	3	The disease is currently active across multiple regions and international borders, and is highly contagious and deadly.

THREAT ASSESSMENT POINTS

THREAT	POINTS	DETAILS
Transmission: Easy	3	Highly infectious. Airborne transmission via tiny water droplets which hang in the air after an infected person coughs or sneezes, long life outside of the human body and picked up on surfaces others touch, contagious, easily spread through casual contact.
Transmission: Moderate	2	Transmission via large water droplets which are temporarily aerosoled by coughing and sneezing, moderate life span on surfaces, spreads through close contact.
Transmission: Difficult	1	Transmission through close contact and prolonged exposure to bodily fluids, short life span outside the body and on surfaces.
Treatment: Easy	1	Either no treatment required or well-established, straightforward treatment protocol relying on easily accessible remedies, little to no antibiotic resistance. Treatment protocol has a proven track record of success.
Treatment: Difficult	2	Complicated or involved treatment protocol using up many resources or rare resources. Pharmaceutical remedies may not be available postdisaster. Treatment protocol does not have a proven track record of success.
Treatment: Lacking	3	There is little to no established treatment protocol. Treatment focuses on palliative care only.
Mortality Rate: 25% or lower	1	Deadly, but odds are generally good if person is healthy, with a strong immune system, no pre-existing chronic conditions, and good nutrition. There may be exceptions to this general rule (for example, Spanish flu pandemic in 1918).
Mortality Rate: 50% or lower	2	Very deadly. Odds of survival are that of a coin toss.
Mortality Rate: Unknown	2	The unknown nature of the disease carries a somewhat higher risk.
Mortality Rate: 75% or lower	3	Exceptionally deadly. Death is the most likely outcome.
Mortality Rate: 100% or lower	4	Unsurvivable given current understanding of the disease and resources.

THREAT ASSESSMENT POINTS		
THREAT	**POINTS**	**DETAILS**
Likelihood of Mutation: Low	1	Certain viruses are less likely to mutate, such as DNA viruses.
Likelihood of Mutation: High	2	RNA viruses are more likely to mutate. Frequency of transmission to new hosts provides more opportunity for mutation. Bacteria are rapidly mutating, developing more virulence and antibiotic resistance.

I also came up with a "watch list." These are diseases that we either currently live with or are not at risk from under current circumstances. But if we were to face a crisis where medications, sanitation, and other modern standards and resources were unavailable, these diseases would spread. Disease always follows disaster.

What Is Threat Level I?

Threat Level I illnesses scored the highest on the Threat Assessment Point Scale (all receiving 11 points), and represent the scenarios which are the most dire. They are easy to transmit through person-to-person contact and lack effective treatments. One, influenza, is a frequently mutating virus that travels the entire globe all year long and predictably reaches the United States every year. Every once in a while, it mutates into something so different from what humans have encountered in the past that we have no natural immunity to it. Another, drug-resistant tuberculosis, recently crossed our border but received precious little press coverage. The final threat in this level, MRSA, and its more serious incarnations as VISA and VRSA, have already spread widely with downplayed importance in the media. Tuberculosis and MRSA are bacteria that have developed strains ranging from resistant to totally resistant against antibiotic drugs. And both influenza and tuberculosis caused multiple pandemics in the past. Influenza, tuberculosis, and MRSA are, in my opinion, the most likely candidates for the next great pandemic.

Influenza

Influenza: deadly strain, with or without cytokine storms

THREAT ASSESSMENT POINTS	
THREAT	POINTS
Past Pandemic	1
Current Epidemic	2
Transmission: Easy	3
Treatment: Lacking	3
Mortality Rate: 25% or lower	1
Bonus points: Mutates easily and frequently	1
TOTAL POINTS	11

Of all of the diseases that might be the next great pandemic, influenza is at the very top of the list. It's the only illness considered here that I felt really deserved a "bonus point" for how often the virus mutates. Because there's always some outbreak of influenza somewhere in the world, moving from the Northern to Southern Hemisphere following colder weather and darker months, it has an unparalleled opportunity to mutate. That deserved some kind of recognition in the rating system.

Influenza has all the makings of a pandemic disaster already in place:
- A solid history of being the repeated cause of a pandemic.
- An easy mode of transmission from person to person.
- An established, cyclical pattern of movement around the globe each year.
- The potential for serious, life-threatening symptoms.
- The ability to mutate, giving rise to new, zoonotic strains to which we have no immunity.

Often simply referred to as "the flu," influenza is an enveloped, RNA virus that has three types: influenza A, influenza B, and influenza C.

Influenza C is rarer than the other two and is more of a problem to dogs and pigs than to humans. Such infections happen once in a while, but tend to be mild.

Influenza B infects humans almost exclusively, but it has been known to infect seals. Influenza B mutates more slowly than influenza A, though it does mutate. We have all had some exposure to previous strains of influenza B and therefore have some level of immunity. But after a few years pass, the virus may finally reach a point where it's genetically new enough that the human body loses that immunity advantage and doesn't fight it off so well. Coming in contact with this strain will give immunity from influenza B for a few more years until it mutates sufficiently again.

While each type of influenza virus is known to infect humans, the type we should be most concerned about is influenza A. This type is known to both mutate more quickly and cause serious infection regularly. It infects people, birds, and swine. Its natural hosts are wild, aquatic birds, such as ducks and geese. Often called avian flu or bird flu even though it also causes infections in pigs and people, it's the most virulent form of influenza.

Being an enveloped, RNA virus, influenza is naturally poised to resist antiviral agents, as well as rapidly and readily mutate. Influenza A strains are categorized by subtype. The subtype refers to two large glycoproteins on the outside of the virus structure, hemagglutinin and neuraminidase. This gives us the H and N in viral subtypes, like H1N1 or H7N9. Research has found 16 H subtypes and 9 N subtypes.

Past Influenza Pandemics. The seasonal flu comes around each year and coincides with when our days get colder and shorter. Each year, there are multiple flu strains present, but one predominant one will emerge. It'll be somewhat different than the year prior. Most years, the flu isn't so bad. Occasionally, we see a rough year where the mutation is so great that humans have little to no natural immunity to the strain. The 2014–15 flu season was one of those years, as was 2009 with the swine flu. While these outbreaks caused a lot of people to be sick, they were minor events compared with the following influenza pandemics:

- 1889–90 Russian flu, killed about 1 million people globally
- 1957 Asian flu, killed about 2 million people globally
- 1968 Hong Kong flu, killed about 500,000 people in Hong Kong

While the 1968 Hong Kong flu spread to other countries, including the United States, the fatalities were fewer than previous outbreaks because of improved medical care and better access to antibiotics for treating secondary infections.

The Deadly Spanish Flu. None of these influenza pandemics came close to the devastation of the Spanish flu of 1918. This pandemic was unique in both the number of people who died and the specific populations who died from it. It's one of the deadliest pandemic events in recorded human history.

To be clear, the Spanish flu was so named because of the amount of media coverage it was permitted in Spain. It didn't originate in Spain, and Spain didn't have more or fewer deaths than anywhere else.

There are several theories of how and where this particular strain of influenza, H1N1, came about. Some think people caught it from local pig or poultry populations, and others claim Chinese soldiers who came to fight in World War I brought it from China. We do know that the virus emerged among soldiers fighting in cramped, close spaces.

This H1N1 influenza virus adapted to seek out a new population: young and healthy adults. This was highly unusual, as influenza is typically more of a threat to the very young, the very old, and those with compromised immune systems. With the Spanish flu, however, it was healthy twenty to fifty year olds (soldiers' age range) with strong immune systems who suffered the most.

The pandemic came in three waves. The first wave started in Kansas. It looked like any other influenza outbreak. The second wave began in August 1918 at three port cities: Boston, United States; Brest, France; and Freeport, Sierra Leone.

The third wave, while not quite as deadly as the second, began in November 1918. The war was over, soldiers were returning home, and the virus traveled with them. In the end, the death toll was staggering: somewhere between 50 and 100 million people dead. The virus spread to the most remote parts of the world, including the Arctic. With potentially a 20 percent mortality rate of those infected, and 3–5 percent of the global population dead, this was hands down one of the deadliest pandemics humankind had ever known.

Why was the Spanish flu outbreak so deadly? Well, the reason for the high death rate has to do with the new segment of the population the virus was targeting. In other flu pandemics, the cause of death is not the flu itself. Instead, it's secondary infections, like bacterial pneumonia in a body that the influenza virus has already weakened. In the Spanish flu, however, in addition to death from secondary infections, there was a new threat in cytokine storms.

Cytokines are a normal part of our body's immune response. They are proteins that help send signals and messages to other cells. They can signal the body's inflammatory response to infection and injury. Normally, the body's feedback will prevent the cytokines from turning into a cytokine storm. In the Spanish flu, that feedback failed to stop the cytokine storm.

Those in that healthy adult demographic with a robust immune system were at a disadvantage here. The cytokine storm was a massive overreaction by their immune system that resulted in hemorrhaging and edema in the lung. They literally died drowning in their own phlegm. The stronger their immune system, the stronger the cytokine storm was.

While pandemic influenza is clearly a risk for a major disaster as the next great pandemic, we need to be aware of its ability to be a major risk after any disaster. In any postdisaster situation, people will be under major stressors, and any influenza infection is more likely to be severe.

Influenza Symptoms and Transmission

Influenza Risk Factors

- Poor ventilation: Sharing space with an infected person, whether or not he or she is still in the room, in places with poor ventilation (close contact not necessary, as influenza is airborne).

- Closed populations: Prisons, hospitals, and nursing homes, and anyone living in crowded conditions with poor ventilation.
- Age: Older and younger populations are at greater risk.
- Compromised immune system: Those with HIV/AIDS, those who have had cancer treatments, those who have had organ transplants, those who suffer from malnutrition, and women who are pregnant are less able to fight off infections like influenza.
- Chronic illness: Raises risk of both infection and complications.
- Hygiene: Lack of adequate hand washing, frequent touching of the face, sharing towels in the bathroom, sharing food or drink with an infected person.

Influenza Symptoms

- Fever of 100°F or higher, sensation of chills
- Nasal congestion
- Cough
- Fatigue
- Sore throat
- Headache/body aches
- Sneezing
- Petechia (little red dots from broken capillaries in face, usually from hard, violent coughing)
- Irritated, red, itchy, watery eyes
- Intestinal discomfort (seen in children)

Influenza has a two-day incubation period from the time a person is infected to when he or she begins to show symptoms. During this time the patient is contagious and can spread the virus to others. The contagious period is usually only up to five days after symptoms begin, but can last up to nine days after symptoms start. This is especially important to remember when in an enclosed population, such as a nursing home, school, or cruise ship.

The three most important symptoms in recognizing influenza are fever, nasal congestion, and cough. When these symptoms last for more than three days and are accompanied by sudden fatigue, it's a good bet that you have the flu and not merely a cold.

Most past influenza pandemics did not include a cytokine storm. A flu can be deadly without causing a cytokine storm, as the Hong Kong,

Asian, and Russian flu pandemics clearly demonstrated. This seems to be the exception, rather than the rule, even when there's an influenza pandemic. Of course, if the next one targets healthy adults with robust immune systems again, then you'll need a way to modulate the cytokine response.

Transmission of the influenza virus happens through the fine water droplets we release when we talk, cough, or sneeze. Because it is aerosoled into the air on those droplets, someone else walking into that area and simply breathing can become infected.

Influenza Response

The best response for every illness on the list is not to get sick in the first place. That can be easier said than done with something so easily transmitted as influenza. But if there's a pandemic flu that becomes active in your area, consider something called a self-imposed reverse quarantine (SIRQ).

A SIRQ is when you voluntarily isolate yourself and the known healthy people in your family or survival group, instead of isolating a sick person. This means no one goes in and no one goes out. If someone goes out, there must be a protocol in place to ensure that the person who leaves the SIRQ can come back in safely, without bringing the virus into the home. Instructions for how to implement a SIRQ are in Chapter 7.

Conventional Medical Response

Conventional medicine doesn't have much to offer when it comes to the flu. Most of the time, the advice given is to stay at home, rest, and drink plenty of fluids. Sometimes, an antiviral influenza medication like Tamiflu is prescribed. If the symptoms become severe and the patient is hospitalized, then he or she may be given oxygen and IV fluids, possibly with prescription expectorants and other symptom medication. But since Tamiflu must be given very early in the infection to be of much use, that leaves oxygen, fluids, and medications. There's still much to be learned about managing cytokine storms, but thankfully, cytokine storms are rarely part of pandemic influenza.

Standard recommendations normally include the following:

- Get plenty of rest.
- Stay well hydrated. This will help to keep the phlegm thinner and easier to expel.
- Take a fever-reducing medication, such as acetaminophen or ibuprofen as needed.
- Stock up on over-the-counter decongestants. Mucinex is what I stock up on as a pharmaceutical expectorant. Its active ingredient is guaifenesin. This is the same medication in Robitussin. But liquids go bad faster than tablets, and tablets avoid that medicinal taste of Robitussin.
- Tamiflu may be prescribed, but it's useful only when prescribed early in the infection.
- If a secondary infection occurs, antibiotics may be prescribed.
- Serious cases may require treatment with oxygen and IV fluids.

Natural and Herbal Response

Use herbal steams frequently. The steams will help soothe the mucous membranes and expel the phlegm. My favorite herb for this is thyme. It's highly antimicrobial and effective on both viral and bacterial respiratory infections. It's also easy to grow. (See sections on tuberculosis and coronavirus for additional ideas on herbal steams, as each of these respiratory ailments is helped with similar herbs and interventions.)

As an alternative or addition, you can add essential oils to herbal steams or use the oils in an aromatherapy diffuser. Lavender and peppermint do a good, gentle job as decongestants. For adults, adding a drop of thyme, eucalyptus, or rosemary oil to the mix is beneficial. Refrain from these oils when treating children. Stick to the safer lavender and peppermint oils until the child is over ten.

Consume lots of soup, preferably made with homemade bone broth. Appropriate herbal additions to this would be ginger, red pepper flakes, garlic, and thyme. This will help keep that mucous running, as well as sooth an irritated throat and sinuses.

Monitor temperature, but refrain from using fever-reducing medications if possible. While this is contrary to standard protocols in conventional medicine, fevers serve a purpose in making the body inhospitable to many pathogens. Fever is a natural immune response. When necessary, opt for diaphoretic herbs (herbs that help induce sweating) as a way to cool a temperature if it's getting too high. Some of my favorite herbs for this purpose with a respiratory infection are garlic, peppermint, and hyssop.

Get as much sunlight as you can without burning. If not possible, take a vitamin D_3 supplement according to package directions.

Address the influenza virus itself. I have found the following remedy, which is based on many of the wonderful suggestions in Stephen Harrod Buhner's book *Herbal Antivirals*, to be extremely helpful:

- 1 ounce of fresh ginger (*Zingiber officinale*) juice
- 5–8 ounces of water (your preference)
- 30 drops of Chinese skullcap (*Scutellaria baicalensis*) tincture
- 30 drops of licorice (*Glycrrhiza glabra*) tincture
- 1 pinch of cayenne (*Capsicum annum*) powder
- 1 tablespoon of raw honey

Juice your ginger, and start heating your water. Add your tinctures and cayenne to the ginger juice. When the water is heated, pour the water into a cup. Then pour the ginger mixture into that cup of water. Sweeten with honey as desired. Take three to four times daily.

In the same book, Buhner also suggests a combination of dong quai (*Angelica sinensis*) and red sage (*Salvia miltiorrhiza*) tinctures in equal amounts, taken in doses of a tablespoon an hour in case of cytokine storms. That's a lot of tincture. If you're going to use this as your backup, make sure to stock a lot of it. At the rate of 1 tablespoon an hour, that's about ⅓ of a quart for just one day. I would plan on having as a backup 3 quarts of this formula prepared ahead of time for one person in case he or she develops a cytokine storm from an influenza viral infection. This would be more than sufficient to cover the needs of a single person for well over a week. If you have four family members, then you need to have 12 quarts. If you're responsible for a larger group of people, you may want to start thinking in gallons. Don't worry; tinctures have a long shelf life.

Use fire cider. Another classic herbal remedy is fire cider, as made famous by the herbalist Rosemary Gladstar. This is a very folksy remedy without measurements. Fill a jar with sliced onions, rough chopped garlic (*Allium sativum*), chopped ginger, chopped horseradish (*Armoracia rusticana*), sliced jalapeños, and a pinch of cayenne powder, and fill to the top with apple cider vinegar. After about two to four weeks, strain everything out and reserve the vinegar. Add some lemon juice and honey. A serving would be 1 ounce. I like to add turmeric (*Curcuma longa*), astragalus (*Astragalus onobrychis*), hibiscus (*Hibiscus sabdariffa*), and sometimes rosemary (*Rosmarinus officinalis*). There are endless variations on Rosemary's original recipe. I prefer to take this by the ounce in an 8-ounce glass of apple juice.

I have my own "instant fire cider" recipe in case you can't wait for two to four weeks. I fill a jar with equal amounts of vinegar, lemon juice, and honey to make 1 cup. To this, I add 1 teaspoon of ginger powder, 1 teaspoon of cayenne powder, ½ teaspoon of turmeric powder, and 1 pinch freshly ground black pepper. Secure the lid to the jar, shake well, and take in teaspoon doses as needed. This is a wonderful herbal decongestant and anti-inflammatory. Adjust the cayenne powder to your heat tolerance. This can be taken as frequently as every fifteen minutes for several hours if necessary.

Make sure that there's good ventilation in the patient's room. If you find that you must enter an area where you suspect the flu virus might be floating about, put a mask on. Look for N95 or P100 respirator masks. These blow out, but do not let air in.

The classic remedy for the flu, however, is elderberry (*Sambucus nigra*). Make it into either a tincture, a glycerite, or a syrup; it doesn't matter. Elderberry is well-known for its effectiveness at treating the flu virus. To make an elderberry tincture, take dried elderberries, fill a jar about three-quarters of the way up with the berries. Fill the rest of the jar with vodka. Let it sit for six weeks, then strain, bottle, and label. Give in doses of 30–60 drops hourly if you suspect the flu. I take my elderberry tincture in a small glass of apple juice daily during cold and flu season to ward off illness.

If the flu progresses and develops a secondary, bacterial pneumonia, you'll need either an herbal or a pharmaceutical antibiotic. Aquatic antibiotics often make an excellent substitution for those marketed to people, provided you get them from the right supplier (see Resources at the end of the book). For pneumonia, options include Fish Mox (amoxicillin 500 mg, three times daily for ten days) and Fish Doxy (doxycycline 100 mg, two times daily for ten days). They're sold in dosages that humans would take. A physician's desk reference will provide you with all the information you need on dosage and frequency of these drugs.

For an herbal alternative, increase the herbal steams. Add juniper (*Juniperus communis*), thyme (*Thymus vulgaris*), sage (*Salvia officinalis*), rosemary, and peppermint (*Mentha piperita*). Sida (*Sida acuta*) tincture, added to the ginger juice cocktail I described above in place of the Chinese skullcap, would be helpful as well.

The last thing I want to mention here is about elderberry and cytokine storms. In a number of places I've read advice from well-meaning people to avoid elderberry at all costs during a pandemic flu, because they believe that it's going to cause a cytokine storm, and the patient will die.

Would that happen? Honestly, I don't know. And neither do any of the other folks already condemning elderberry as a big "no no" for cytokine storms. Elderberry does have some ability to increase cytokine action. But it also has some actions that may help keep those cytokines in check. There's just no real way to know other than to try it out. But that would require an actual cytokine storm to find out, which is usually an emergency situation and hard to come by in a clinical test setting.

Another option is to make a tea or tincture of elderflowers. I have found these to be both gentle and effective at helping respiratory complaints from mild asthma and allergies to congestion common to the flu.

To reiterate, not all pandemic influenza outbreaks result in cytokine storms. Odds are, the cytokine storm is a moot point, since influenza pandemics are common and cytokine storms with them are not. Take your elderberry tincture, fight the flu, and don't worry about it. But if cytokine storms as caused by that particular strain, cease taking the elderberry and see the above recommendations for cytokine storms.

Tuberculosis

THREAT ASSESSMENT POINTS	
THREAT	POINTS
Past Pandemic	1
Current Pandemic	2
Transmission: Moderate	2
Treatment: Lacking	3
Mortality Rate: 75% or lower	3
TOTAL POINTS	11

Tied for first place with influenza is tuberculosis, which is caused by bacteria called *Mycobacterium tuberculosis*. The shorthand is M. tuberculosis (or even shorter, TB). M. tuberculosis can spread throughout the body via the bloodstream and the lymphatic system, growing nodules called tubercles along the way. The bacteria prefers, however, to attack the lungs. This is called pulmonary tuberculosis. This is the most common form, and the type covered here.

When a person is infected with M. tuberculosis, this doesn't mean he or she will automatically develop the disease state we call tuberculosis. When a person inhales the M. tuberculosis bacteria into the lung, the immune system is almost always sufficient to respond to the threat. But the way our immune system responds to M. tuberculosis is analogous to putting the bacteria in a type of "jail cell" as opposed to killing it. Infected people will not have any symptoms and may never even know that they're infected. This is what's known as latent tuberculosis, or latent TB.

In fact, 90 percent of all patients infected will have latent tuberculosis, while 10 percent of patients will develop symptoms known as active tuberculosis, or active TB. For someone who has latent TB, if the immune system becomes weakened or stressed, it may not be sufficient to keep the bacteria in "jail" any longer. At this point, the infection is known as active TB. The person will develop symptoms and become very sick. Left untreated, tuberculosis has a mortality rate of 50 percent. Chances of survival are greatly increased, however, when tuberculosis is diagnosed and treated with effective antibiotics early.

Where a typical viral or bacterial infection might call for a course of antibiotics lasting ten to fourteen days, standard tuberculosis care requires a course of multiple antibiotics, which typically lasts six to nine months, and often much longer. This has become far more complicated with the development of drug-resistant tuberculosis (DR-TB), multidrug-resistant tuberculosis (MDR-TB), extensively drug-resistant tuberculosis (XDR-TB), and finally, totally drug-resistant tuberculosis (TDR-TB).

Without the presence of antibiotic resistance, tuberculosis remains active and contagious for a minimum of two to three weeks while antibiotics are initially given to the patient. This contagious period may be considerably longer depending on whether the strain is resistant to antibiotics, and if so, how resistant.

India has been particularly hard hit by tuberculosis. While WHO spends time trying to decide on the parameters for the definition of TDR-TB, people are dying without proper screening. While I appreciate the need for standards and specificity, in the real world everyone knows what "totally drug-resistant tuberculosis" means: there's no antibiotic that will cure you if you're infected with TDR-TB. You're only slightly less in trouble if you have XDR-TB. At least, there's still a chance for antibiotic treatments to work, though they may require a person to take antibiotics for twice as long. The more antibiotics that tuberculosis outsmarts, the more at risk all of humanity is.

The Advent of Totally Drug-Resistant Tuberculosis. There are several factors driving the increase in drug-resistant tuberculosis. The first is that TB is common in very poor populations. Tuberculosis is quite active in Central and South Americas, Africa, India, the Middle

East, Eastern European nations, Russia, and most of Asia. Many of these areas are poverty-stricken and lack the deep pockets to pay for drugs, and are therefore unattractive to pharmaceutical companies.

Another connection to poverty, in poor areas, is that there is very little testing done to verify if an infection is TB or something else. Antibiotics are given straight away in case it's tuberculosis. This leads to many patients being given unnecessary antibiotics because most doctors won't risk not prescribing them just in case it's not just the flu. Just as there's little testing of the patient for TB, there's even less testing for the specific strain of TB, and therefore no way to know which antibiotic drugs would be the most effective without contributing to more antibiotic resistance.

Tuberculosis is something most Americans just don't think about. To most of us, tuberculosis is an affliction of a bygone era. Once known as "consumption" and "the white plague," tuberculosis has become an infection of the past thanks to antibiotics, at least to our first-world minds. Some of our grandparents who entered the United States through Ellis Island may remember immigration officials putting people into quarantine if they looked sick. One of the primary diseases immigration officials screened for was tuberculosis. But for recent generations, tuberculosis is simply not something we think about in the United States. Perhaps we should.

The Current Global Tuberculosis Pandemic. Most people in the United States are blissfully unaware that there's a current tuberculosis pandemic active right now. You won't find many stories on the evening news about it. While the words "global tuberculosis pandemic" may be hard to find, statistics on tuberculosis are not. According to both CDC and WHO, over one-third of the global population is infected with TB. Let that sink in a moment. At least 33 percent of the global population has been infected with *Mycobacterium tuberculosis*. At the time of this writing (October 2015), using the estimated current population from two "world clocks" at www.WorldoMeters.info and www.census.gov of over 7 billion people (I approximated their running totals and used 7,246,164,000 for my calculations), and one-third of this is just shy of 2.5 billion people.

From there, we can extrapolate an approximate number for the current total of latent TB and active TB cases globally. The latent TB patients would be 90 percent of 2.5 billion, which is 2.25 billion. The active TB patients would be the remaining 10 percent, which is 250 million. These numbers are important, as they provide the "big picture" view of tuberculosis. This is already a deadly pandemic that has crossed international borders. It is kept at bay only by antibiotics. As the bacteria develops more drug resistance, it'll become a much deadlier pandemic than it already is.

Knowing the global totals helps put other statistics in perspective. CDC and WHO both report that there were about 9 million people who became sick with tuberculosis in 2013. That doesn't mean that there were only 9 million people who were sick globally; rather, this represents new cases of active tuberculosis. This includes those who were newly infected as well as those who had latent TB, which became active TB. Still, this is a subset of the total active cases.

The total global population in 2013 was approximately 7.2 billion, according to a United Nations press release in June 2013 on population increase and projections. Since the 2013 data are the latest information published on the websites and are only somewhat smaller than the current population figures I have used here in 2015 of 7.246 billion, the 9 million figure from 2013 is still a useful and relevant figure.

Reporting that there were only 9 million new cases of active TB is much less alarming than reporting something like, "Of the total 250 million current, active cases, 9 million are new cases." While this isn't technically "underreporting," it's picking and choosing statistics that may give people a rosier picture of the global tuberculosis status.

Tuberculosis and US Politics. Looking at statistics specifically for our own country, in March 2015 CDC had 9,421 active cases of tuberculosis reported in the United States.[14] In this report, it brags that this is a decrease of 2.2 percent. To put this in perspective, the total

_____
14 http://www.cdc.gov/mmwr/preview/mmwrhtml/mm6410a2.htm.

new active cases reported by CDC from 2013 is 9,582.[15] We're talking only a difference of 161 cases.

This total is further broken down into tuberculosis patients who are US-born persons and foreign-born persons. A 66.5 percent majority of active cases reported in the United States in 2014 were in foreign-born patients, and a very slight increase from 65 percent in 2013. Furthermore, 90 percent of all cases of MDR-TB came from foreign-born patients.

This is where the threat of tuberculosis takes an interesting turn. We now have a political agenda intersecting with a viable threat of MDR-TB. This was plainly the case in 2014's immigration crisis when tens of thousands of children and adults crossed multiple international borders to reach the United States and overwhelmed our border patrol's capacity to properly screen those coming into the United States.

This was a politically divisive issue, as all American political discourse is, with each side of the political aisle pandering to its core constituency. If you showed compassion for the children, you would be called out as a bleeding heart liberal. If you showed any concern for the reports of adult, male gang members among the refugee children, or if you showed concern over reports that these refugees were bringing in scabies, measles, and tuberculosis, then you were a heartless conservative. So, bleeding heart versus heartless. Perhaps we should leave emotion and political maneuvering at the door.

Events like a mass exodus of tens of thousands of children and young adults from Central and South America walking through jungles and crossing several national boundaries don't just happen within a vacuum. This crisis came about through a mixture of gang violence, overwhelming poverty, and our own policies for children entering the United States illegally, but without an adult.

In 2008 then-president George W. Bush signed the William Wilberforce Trafficking Victims Protection Reauthorization Act. This law was intended to provide a measure of protection for minors, from countries not bordering the United States, who were here illegally, and without a parent or legal guardian. The reasoning was that these

15 http://www.cdc.gov/tb/statistics.

children may very well have been sold into the slave or sex trade, and a hearing was needed to determine if it was safe to return them to their country of origin, or if we would simply be sending them back to people who would turn around and sell them again.

The problem with this is the court system has become overwhelmed, and these hearings end up severely delayed. Many minors turn eighteen here in the United States before a hearing can be held. In effect, if a child from a country not bordering the United States were to come here alone, he or she would be unlikely to be deported. While that's not the official policy, in practice, this is what the policy has become. In the time they're here, however, they're placed with families, attend school, and make a life for themselves. Mexican children are not included in this act and therefore do not receive the same treatment.

This has become extremely appealing to desperate parents. Families in countries like El Salvador, Honduras, and Guatemala desperately hand over their life savings to smugglers, known as coyotes, to smuggle their children into the United States in hopes of a better life. The coyote may honor the agreement and indeed smuggle the child as safely as possible across our border. But it's just as likely that the coyote may sell the child or abandon the child if the situation becomes dangerous.

As the violence in Central America has grown and continues to grow, and the belief that the United States "isn't deporting children" spreads, the number of coyotes escorting children has increased into the tens of thousands. This has allowed cover for a more violent and criminal element to hide among these children. To make matters worse, there's no effective way to track these individuals once placed with care providers.

While we have a policy that in theory says we deport but in practice invites children to stay, we shouldn't be surprised that children began actually showing up. Policymakers should have foreseen this. Unfortunately, there were no accommodations; people of all ages were sleeping on the floor in cramped spaces. Stories surfaced about the scabies, chicken pox, measles, and tuberculosis that the US Border Patrol was faced with from these children. These infections are far more common in Central America, and it isn't hard to see how under these less-than-ideal circumstances, infections and disease have a chance to spread. Rumors began to circulate in the media of gag orders on nurses and other care providers working in these holding facilities. Reports of young children and adults being relocated around the country began leaking into the media.

More than one governor was surprised to learn only after the fact that these children had been relocated within their state borders, including my home state of Massachusetts. Eyewitnesses reported border-crossing children and adults being transported to Massachusetts by plane, brought to Hanscom Air Force Base, and then put on buses to destinations unknown. Then-governor Deval Patrick had made a public statement that no such children were being housed here, only to find out a day or two later that, in fact, there were children being relocated to homes in Massachusetts and New Hampshire.[16] This was likely to avoid having to contend with protesters, but the lack of transparency did not help an already contentious situation.

Politicians would much rather turn this into a political issue, working voters into a lather to boost numbers at the polls rather than address it as a medical one. It was a great example of political pandering on both sides, how politicians and the media take every opportunity to be divisive, and how such shortsightedness can take a poorly handled immigration crisis and turned it into a full-blown pandemic nightmare.

What we can learn from this is the following:

- Tuberculosis is still a threat in the United States.
- While we have several thousand cases in the United States each year, the threat most frequently enters the United States from other countries where tuberculosis, and drug-resistant tuberculosis, is more common.
- Ignoring the problem is not going to make it go away.
- Politicians and mainstream media are more likely to take the opportunity to exploit the situation to further their careers than to address the problem.

---

16 http://www.unionleader.com/apps/pbcs.dll/article?AID=/20140612/NEWS06/140619533/0/news03.

- Politicians will use the media to push their agenda, and that takes priority over health and well-being.
- You cannot have any expectation of transparency from the government during a crisis, especially one it helped create.

And while the border crisis may present a risk for tuberculosis cases, we live in a world where people are welcome to travel in our country. We have tourists, families from overseas, exchange students, researchers, and even some that are not here through legal channels, who fly into our airports and drive or walk across our borders every day. If a disease exists "out there" in a foreign country, it can exist "in here," within our borders. As time goes on, and people travel, and drug resistance increases, a deadly outbreak of totally drug-resistant tuberculosis will be an even greater threat to become the next great pandemic.

I would also caution people that since tuberculosis is already here, TB would be a major threat not only as a disaster in and of itself but also a disease to be on the lookout for if we have a disaster of another kind.

Tuberculosis Symptoms and Transmission

Tuberculosis Risk Factors
- Compromised immune system: Those with HIV/AIDS, those who have had cancer treatments, those who have had organ transplants, those who suffer from malnutrition, and women who are pregnant are less able to fight off infections like influenza.
- Chronic disease: Such as diabetes and liver or kidney disease.
- Lack of adequate hospital staff to provide health care regularly for TB patients: Pandemics and economics push hospital staff and resources to their limits.
- Closed populations: Prisons, hospitals, and nursing homes, and anyone living in crowded conditions with poor ventilation.
- Travel to areas known for tuberculosis: India, China, Russia, Pakistan, sub-Saharan Africa, and Central America.

Pulmonary tuberculosis starts out similar to a flu, with fever, chills, and coughing. In both cases, appetites may be suppressed. But one of the major differences is in the duration of illness. The flu is usually over within a couple of weeks. If symptoms, such as a deep cough, persist beyond two to three weeks, it's time to start suspecting other causes than influenza. This could be a secondary bacterial infection, like bronchitis or pneumonia. It could be a fungal respiratory infection. Or, it could be tuberculosis.

Tuberculosis Symptoms

- Severe cough
- Duration of illness three weeks or longer
- Coughing up blood-tinged sputum
- Fever and chills
- Fatigue
- Muscle weakness
- Sore throat
- Distinct loss of appetite leading to weight loss
- Night sweats

Another important symptom to watch for is blood in the phlegm (a.k.a., mucus, sputum). Tuberculosis will produce a yellow phlegm with evidence of blood in it. This is from the painful, violent coughing. This is not proof of TB, as it could also be anything from acute bronchitis to cancer. But it may also be tuberculosis.

Tuberculosis spreads much the same way that influenza spreads. TB is found in the small water droplets that are transmitted through the air, person to person, by coughing, sneezing, speaking, or singing. I list "singing" for the sake of completeness, as this mode of transmission is taken directly from CDC's website.[17] It must be somewhat painful to sing with tuberculosis, but I'm sure the positive outlook is helpful.

It's possible to get tuberculosis by sharing food and drink, but it's not the most common way to get it. The easiest way to become infected with TB is to inhale the bacteria in the air when someone has recently coughed or sneezed in that air space.

Transmission takes place most easily where people are in cramped locations and within enclosed populations. Examples of enclosed populations include schools, dormitories, nursing homes, hospitals,

---

17 http://www.cdc.gov/tb/topic/basics.

and prisons. A single person infected with TB on a crowded subway train could infect ten to fifteen people easily by coughing.

At the beginning of the Industrial Era, tuberculosis was rampant in England. Entire families would work in factories, come home to eat and sleep, and get ready to do it all again the next day. To save on money, multiple families rented apartments together. When one family was at the factory, the other was at home, sleeping, eating, bathing, and so forth. The families slept in shifts, coughing into their pillows, never changing out the bed linens before the next person got into bed. The apartments were small, and through coughing and sneezing, the apartment became filled with M. tuberculosis for the other family to breathe into their lungs.

Without an effective antibiotic treatment, the mortality rate in tuberculosis patients is above 50 percent. Cramped, enclosed spaces, without much fresh air, most often without proper rest or nutrition, led to many TB infections.

Tuberculosis Response

If there's an outbreak in your area, please consider a SIRQ. While this could be said about each illness mentioned in this book, it's especially important for tuberculosis. TB is a long-haul disease. If you get it, you're not going to be well again for perhaps a year or longer, weakness lingers long after recovery, and the resources you have to have stockpiled to see you through this kind of disaster are significant.

Let's assume that you do become ill with tuberculosis. Do you have enough food to feed yourself until you're well? True, your appetite will decrease. That's why it was once known as consumption. The person was being consumed by the disease and shrinking away to nothingness, leaving only a frail, weak shell behind. At least having your home-canned and dehydrated foods will keep the energy output to simply reheating and rehydrating. Do you have enough, however, to see you through to a full recovery?

Do you have a water source that will allow you to have running water and indoor plumbing in case public utilities fail? If they do, does your method/source require labor? If so, who will do the labor? If you have tuberculosis, it's not going to be you.

The same question must also be applied to other necessities, like cooking and heating fuel, child care if you have small children, and a major one: do you have enough cash in the bank to cover your expenses while you're ill? Even if society itself does not collapse, but is only pushed really hard, so to speak, if you have TB, you're not going to work. You also cannot rely on unemployment or sick time or vacation time or short-term disability to cover you either. Think of how many other people will be drawing on those same resources. Even if they qualify, everyone will get the runaround with denial after denial because the funds will run out.

OK, deep breath (but not around anyone with tuberculosis): let's look at how modern medicine approaches TB care and what we can learn from it.

Conventional Medical Response

The modern treatment protocol for tuberculosis relies on antibiotic drugs, which do not have an aquatic antibiotic equivalent. This is not something for which you can stock up on Fish Mox and call yourself prepared. The antibiotics being used for tuberculosis, not taking into account any drug resistance, include the following:

- Isoniazid
- Rifampin (Rifadin, Rimactane)
- Ethambutol (Myambutol)
- Pyrazinamide

These are then used together for six to nine months. If there's drug resistance, some of the following may be added to treatment:

- Fluoroquinolones
- Amikacin
- Kanamycin
- Capreomycin

Because these are uncommon and don't have an aquatic equivalent, in the event of a tuberculosis pandemic, you're not going to have access to these unless you go to a hospital. But I would expect the antibiotics that are still effective against TB to run out, and run out quickly. I expect that there will be some movement of supply and hoarding by medical facilities and the government. After every document that I have checked on the Strategic National Stockpile, I cannot find any evidence that these specific antibiotics are being stockpiled.

This leaves us to look at how the medical community handled TB cases prior to antibiotics, what worked from that, and what did not. In addition, there are herbal medicines and practical steps that may be of some use. CDC recommends PPE for health care providers working with TB patients, especially an N95 mask. I prefer the P100 masks because the filters are refillable and last longer. It's also advisable to use other basic PPE, such as protective gloves. Another simple recommendation is to set up the sickroom with negative air pressure. In other words, set up a window fan to blow the air out.

Natural and Herbal Response

How was tuberculosis treated before antibiotics? In the United States, it was in facilities known as sanatoriums. Not to be confused with sanitarium, a sanatorium was a facility that took care of people with long-term illnesses. While many died in these facilities, if a person was admitted early in the disease, sanatoriums did well by their patients. The protocol for TB patients rested on two primary goals:

1. Rest: absolute rest. More rest than one can imagine.
2. Plenty of well-ventilated, fresh air.

Patients who sought treatment would literally lie in bed, getting up for only the most basic of functions, such as going to the toilet and sitting on the edge of the bed with a basin for bathing. But as time went on, activity was increased ever so slowly. The patient was then allowed to sit up for an hour each day. These incremental changes from week to week permitted the body the space it needed to fight off the disease. It took great discipline to rest as much as was necessary for as long as was necessary.

People would be separated from their family and friends for six months to a year while the nursing and medical staff saw to their every need. This is not to say it was a luxurious stay with gourmet meals or anything, but there was nothing to do but rest and let the body heal itself. A detailed record of life in a sanatorium can be found in the

Journal of the Royal Society of Medicine.[18] It's a diary of a woman who became sick with active TB. She details her concerns, the reality of living in a sanatorium, the attitude she cultivated there, and how she recovered. She went on to live a full life, having a second child, and dying in her eighties of natural causes.

Reading her diary entry provides some insight on how you might establish a sickroom and your own group's tuberculosis protocols for care.

Establish a sickroom with negative pressure. A window-fan blowing air outside works well.

Patient commits himself or herself to bed rest only. Complete bed rest was a key part of successful tuberculosis care in sanatoriums.

Focus on nutritionally dense food. Patient will lose appetite, so make every bite count. Potentially, supplement with a multivitamin.

Make an herbal tincture. This tincture supports your immune system while it tackles the TB. Use equal amounts of the following herbs in a jar with vodka, and allow to steep for six weeks. Strain, bottle, and label. Toss the old plant material. Use a standard dosage and frequency, three to four times per day with 1 dropperful in a small glass of water.

• Astragalus
• Rhodiola (*Rhodiola rosea*)
• Sida (*Sida acuta*)
• Sweet Annie (*Artemisia annua*)

Herbal steams. There are some herbs with antibiotic actions, but they must come in contact with the tissue for it to work. These are considered local antibiotic herbs. Others are systemic, such as *Sida acuta* and Sweet Annie, and will travel with the blood throughout the body. The use of herbal steams brings that herb directly to the infected tissue. To make an herbal steam, boil a pot of water on the stove, take it off the heat (and place on a trivet to prevent it damaging anything), add your herbs, maybe a tablespoon of each, and drape a towel over your head and face, tenting it over the pot of steaming herbs. Be careful not to get burned by the steam. Make an herbal steam out of any or all of the following:

18 http://www.ncbi.nlm.nih.gov/pmc/articles/PMC1079536.

- Thyme leaf
- Juniper berry
- Rosemary
- Lavender (*Lavandula officinalis*)
- Red pepper flake (*Capsicum annum*)
- Sage leaf
- Peppermint

Make an herbal expectorant tea. Allow a cup of hot water to steep some of the following herbs, covered, for twenty minutes before drinking, then add honey:

- Hyssop (*Hyssopus officinalis*)
- Licorice
- Clove (*Syzygium aromaticum*)
- Elecampane (*Inula helenium*)
- Coltsfoot (*Tussilago farfara*)

Make good use of demulcent herbs. These herbs produce a thick, slippery texture in water and help encourage moistening of our mucous membranes. To do this, my favorite option it to make a cold infusion of marshmallow (*Althaea officinalis*), and I include cinnamon (*Cinnamomum burmannii*) chips for flavor. Sometimes I might grab some peppermint from my yard instead of the cinnamon, and it works beautifully. To make a cold infusion, get a quart-sized mason jar, fill it one-quarter of the way full with marshmallow root, add in one-quarter of a cup of cinnamon chips, and then pour room temperature water over the marshmallow in the jar. Allow this to steep on the counter for a minimum of four hours, maximum overnight. Strain out the plant material, and drink the liquid. It doesn't need to be consumed all at once, but sip it periodically throughout the day.

Triple It. Whatever guideline you use to stock up on the essentials like food, water, and money to pay bills during the interim, you should triple it to make sure that you're covered.

Staphylococcus Aureas (MRSA, VISA, and VRSA)

THREAT ASSESSMENT POINTS	
THREAT	**POINTS**
Current Epidemic	2
Transmission: Easy	2
Treatment: Lacking	3
Mortality Rate Depends on type of infection (MRSA-2, VISA-3, and VRSA-4) and how far the infection has progressed. For example, when a skin infection of MRSA is treated early, there's little risk of a fatality. But left untreated, MRSA has the opportunity to move deeper in the body, and it can cause septicemia, with a 30 percent mortality rate.	2–4
TOTAL POINTS	9–11

Staphylococcus aureas is a gram-positive bacteria that is actually part of our normal, human flora. Both S. aureas and S. epidermidis can be nonpathogenic, meaning that they do not lead to disease and help us fight off nonindigenous bacteria. But when staphylococcus grows out of control, that's when we have problems. S. aureas is more likely to grow out of control and therefore tends to cause more problems than S. epidermidis.

Pathogenic S. aureus is typically found in skin infections, in the respiratory system's mucous membranes, and infected foods. Once in the body, it can spread throughout nearly any tissue. Once infected, S. aureus releases exotoxins. Which toxins are released depends on the strain of S. aureas. These exotoxins can result in toxic shock syndrome (TSS), staphylococcal scalded skin syndrome (SSSS), and necrotizing (flesh-eating) pneumonia.

S. aureas is typically treated with some form of the antibiotic penicillin, such as for a sinus infection. But strains of S. aureas have developed powerful, thorough, and effective resistance mechanisms to penicillin and related antibiotics. In the case of MRSA (methicillin-resistant S. aureas), methicillin is a narrow-spectrum antibiotic drug that has been very effective on S. aureas in the past. The bacteria's adaptability, however, has created strains resistant to it and other powerful antibiotics. It would be fair to say that calling these strains methicillin-resistant is a gross understatement.

When most people think of drug-resistant bacteria, MRSA is almost always what they think of first. But MRSA isn't the only drug-resistant bacteria that poses a threat. Just like TDR-TB, there are several other bacteria with drug resistance, which one could make a reasonable argument for being the next great pandemic, such as E. coli, as well as both *Salmonella typhi* and nontyphoidal salmonella, *Clostridium difficile*, and *Klebsiella pneumoniae*. C. difficile and K. pneumoniae are deadly bacteria that are commonly acquired in a hospital setting. C. difficile and K. pneumoniae are even more difficult to treat. In CDC's "Antibiotic Resistance Threats Report" from 2013, both C. difficile and K. pneumoniae are listed as threat level "Urgent," more dire than MRSA at threat level "Serious." MRSA stands apart from them for two reasons:

1. MRSA escaped the hospital.

2. MRSA has developed both a nearly totally drug-resistant strain, vancomycin-intermediate *Staphylococcus aureas* (VISA), and a totally drug-resistant strain, vancomycin-resistant *Staphylococcus aureas* (VRSA).

MRSA was once strictly a hospital-acquired infection. But this bacteria has evolved and escaped from the hospital. Community-acquired MRSA is increasingly common. MRSA illness from our food supply has occurred, but remains a little-discussed threat. Airborne MRSA infections are even less discussed, but still happen. To begin to understand the MRSA threat, we have to recognize its adaptability to spread.

Where K. pneumoniae may be closer to having more total drug resistance than MRSA (not counting VISA infections), it's still a hospital-acquired bacteria. Where salmonella may be in every chicken and egg at the grocery store, as well as on the grocery store shelves and shopping cart, it's still a food-borne bacteria. *Neisseria gonorrhoeae*, the bacteria that causes gonorrhea, is a sexually transmitted, community-acquired bacteria that is also more resistant to drug therapy than MRSA.

MRSA, on the other hand, has crossed all barriers. It's hospital acquired, community acquired, food acquired, and sometimes even sexually transmitted. MRSA is in every hospital, doctor's office, and nursing facility. It's in the community, often found in locker rooms, schools, military bases, jails, stadiums, theaters, shopping malls, and anywhere there are crowded people.

VISA infections are, thankfully, less common. They remain, for the time being, hospital-acquired infections. Given the extraordinary ease with which bacteria communicate, it's only a matter of time before more staph infections are VRSA and VISA infections, including community-acquired infections.

While any drug-resistant bacteria could pose a threat to a community, MRSA stands out. Combining the ever-growing antibiotic resistance of MRSA with its ease of transmission, this strikes me as a far greater risk for a pandemic than some other drug-resistant bacterial infections that have remained behind hospital walls.

The dangers of contracting MRSA are serious. MRSA can move beyond the initial infected site to the body's soft tissues. Life-threatening infections can move from either a wound or a boil deep into bones and joints. MRSA can also travel through the bloodstream, to the heart valves. While MRSA is most often found in the skin flora, it's also found in the nose and can travel to the lungs as well.

One interesting thing about the MRSA pandemic is that the most common place to contract it is in a hospital. MRSA is one of those reasons to avoid going to a hospital or medical facility unless it's absolutely necessary. If you had surgery or went in with an open wound, both two very common occurrences for a hospital, you could easily get MRSA. If you simply breathe the air in a hospital, you might get MRSA.

As more staph bacteria learn and adapt, and more staph infections are VRSA and VISA infections, we will have very little defense against them. This would make for plausible and probable pandemic. As VISA spread, a significant percentage of everyone who entered a hospital would ultimately become infected. This new level of drug-resistance would spread to community-acquired infections, and then quickly spread among high school and college athletics programs, dormitories, prisons, military training facilities, hotels, train and bus stations, amusement parks, and anywhere that people get injured, are in close quarters, or congregate in large numbers.

MRSA/VISA/VRSA Symptoms and Transmission

MRSA/VISA/VRSA Risk Factors

- Having been in a hospital, doctor's office, walk-in clinic, same-day surgical center, dialysis center, nursing home, or other medical facility.
- Had a medical procedure, such as a surgery, had a medical device implanted, or had any kind of medical tubing (e.g., intravenous line, catheter) inserted.
- Having been in a prison, dormitory, locker room, child care facility, or other crowded space, especially where sanitation may be an issue.
- Having been to a gym, played contact sports, been in competition (e.g., obstacle races or military training facilities), or any situation where there's contact with other people and a high risk of getting an abrasion or cut.

MRSA/VISA/VRSA Symptoms

A staphylococcal infection of the skin may present as small, red bumps that progress into a boil. These red bumps may also resemble, at first, minor acne, a spider bite, or mosquito bites, but will develop into a pus-filled boil. With MRSA, that boil will quickly increase in size and can be several inches in diameter. There will be pain, heat, and redness, which are clear signs of infection. This can also develop in any cut or open wound. Ultimately, MRSA's impact will be tissue death, or necrosis, wherever it infects.

Common infections associated with MRSA are urinary tract infections (UTIs), sinus infections, and pharyngitis. The problems begin, however, when the bacteria move deeper into the body. When MRSA infects the bones and joints, when it reaches the blood and travels to the organs and heart, this is when MRSA becomes a deadly threat. MRSA can lead to septicemia and sepsis, an abscess in the brain or in the spinal column, cellulitis, pneumonia, kidney failure, and endocarditis.

MRSA/VISA/VRSA Transmission

To be clear, transmission of MRSA is very easy. It's transmitted to people from surfaces, from contact with other people, through the food supply, through sex, and by breathing it in.[19, 20]

If MRSA is on a surface or on another person, it is highly contagious. MRSA can be spread on fabric, such as shared bed linens with an infected person. If there's an open wound, there's an even greater chance of becoming infected. If MRSA is in the air, and you decide to take a nice deep breath of hospital air, there's a risk of infection. Any facility that recirculates air is possibly spreading MRSA throughout the building.

Along with E. coli, salmonella, and listeria, MRSA is found in our food supply. It remains in the environment around the factory farm,[21] tripling the risk of everyone within a mile of the factory farm of becoming infected with MRSA. In 2012 a research paper titled "Methicillin-Resistant Staphylococci: Implications for Our Food Supply,"[22] detailed 240,000 illnesses related to heat-resistant enterotoxins caused by S. aureas that occur in the United States annually, and how resistant strains further complicate the matter. Recently, MRSA was found in two-thirds of pork products in Denmark. Finally, MRSA has been transmitted during sexual contact. This has occurred through both oral sex and intercourse.[23] But it can just as easily be spread by sharing the same bed linens.[24] So, technically, it's not a sexually transmitted disease, because it can be spread other ways than through sexual contact. But,

---

19 http://www.ncbi.nlm.nih.gov/pubmed/11405862.
20 http://courses.washington.edu/cee490/MRSAWP.htm.
21 http://archinte.jamanetwork.com/article.aspx?articleid=1738717.
22 http://www.ncbi.nlm.nih.gov/pubmed/23253164.
23 https://ispub.com/IJID/8/2/6466.
24 http://cid.oxfordjournals.org/content/44/12/1664.1.full.

as a practical matter, this is probably splitting hairs. Bottom line, MRSA could be anywhere.

MRSA/VISA/VRSA Response

If MRSA were to develop into a VISA pandemic, where would you seek treatment? Would you go to a hospital? What kind of treatment could the hospital offer when even vancomycin fails? Hospitals are where most patients become exposed to MRSA in the first place. So, if it got that bad, would medical staff even show up to work in a facility where just being in the building may very well expose them, and by extension their families, to a VISA or VRSA infection?

Would a completely different type of facility be opened to treat such infections? Would an outdoor area be better for MRSA treatment as opposed to an indoor treatment center with recirculating air? And without effective antibiotics, what would patients receive as treatment?

Once the magnitude of a VISA pandemic was acknowledged, few people would want to go to the hospital for anything. Not only would you need to be ready to deal with MRSA, VISA, or VRSA, but there would be a host of other medical situations arguing against the necessity of an ER visit.

Conventional Medical Response. For treatment of drug-resistant staph infections, conventional medicine depends on the development of new antibiotics. The absolute last line of defense that conventional medicine currently has, short of amputating an infected limb, is a class of drugs called "streptogramins." If these don't work, then nothing is going to work to stop the infection from spreading through the body.

This presents those who are concerned about medical preparedness with two problems.

- There is no "vet med" antibiotic equivalent to streptogramins.
- Streptogramins are administered intravenously. This requires more skill than the average household will have.

Natural and Herbal Response. As an herbalist, I'm biased toward using herbal medicine. But I would strongly urge anyone preparing for a pandemic, or any type of disaster where access to medicine may be cut off, to learn how to use herbs for their therapeutic benefits. In the case of MRSA, learning how to make and create herbal remedies with antibiotic properties could save your life.

While bacteria are some of the oldest forms of life on earth, plants have also been around for a long time. Plants, like bacteria, evolve. Where bacteria have developed defense mechanisms, plants have developed their own. Unlike a pharmaceutical antibiotic drug, which is formulated and then replicated in the exact same manner each and every time, allowing bacteria to adapt to them completely, bacteria have not developed a corresponding resistance to botanical antibiotic remedies.

The other aspect of plant-based medicines that give them an edge over antibiotic drugs is that plants are complex synergies of chemical constituents. Pharmaceutical drugs rely on individual active ingredients. This is much easier for bacteria to understand and defeat. Herbs present a far more complex problem to the bacteria.

While most mainstream medical organizations downplay the effectiveness of herbal medicines or default to the tired claim that there's a lack of evidence to support the claims that herbal formulas work, there are new studies done every year demonstrating exactly that. This is true even where herbs and MRSA are concerned. Please do not let professional protectionism deter you from making an informed choice about herbal medicines and their effectiveness.

Skin Infections. This type of MRSA infection can frequently be handled without taking antibiotic drugs, but not always. A lot depends on how early it's treated and how efficient the patient's immune system is. Normally, a doctor will make an incision and carefully drain out the pus with gloved fingers. This is painful—much more painful than dealing with a normal boil and over a much larger area, but very necessary. There's often a hard core resembling a cyst that may come out as well. Once completely drained, there's often an open wound left where the pus and the hard core once was. If this is the case, the wound will need to be packed with gauze, treated with some kind of antibacterial agent, cleaned regularly, and watched closely as it heals.

If you attempt to drain the boil for someone in your group, be sure to wear PPE at all times during the procedure. Wear gloves, face mask, goggles, and gown. If possible, do this indoors, in a room with negative air pressure (fan blowing out the window). The pus can spurt and splatter. Be very careful to avoid contact with it.

Once you've drained the boil and the wound is open and empty, my choice would be to fill it with honey-soaked gauze. A study was done on multiple types of honey, including buckwheat, blueberry, clover, and Manuka honey, among many honeys, testing their effectiveness against MRSA. All the various honeys were found effective against MRSA, owing to honey's ability to manufacture small amounts of hydrogen peroxide at the site of the infection continually.[25]

Honey is one of the best natural remedies for skin infections and open wounds that you can have on hand. Not only is it effective, it has an indefinite shelf life. If it begins to crystallize, you can warm it back up (no higher than 115°F), and it will reliquefy like it came fresh from the hive. You can order raw honey online in 5-gallon buckets from beekeeping supply companies, such as Brushy Mountain Bee Farm. But the best way to secure a honey source is to raise your own bees. Otherwise, get very friendly with a local beekeeper. After a disaster hits, the local beekeeper will suddenly get very popular. Honey is one of the most valuable things you can stockpile. It's used in medicine, food preservation, food preparation, and skin care. I would strongly urge you to keep your own hives.

Honey can be enhanced with botanicals by steeping herbs in it. Herbs that would be of use to skin infections would be garlic,[26] ginger,[27] Oregon grape root, or any herb containing the chemical berberine.[28] Fill a jar with the herb of your choice and cover it with honey. Leave to steep for a couple of weeks, or you can use a Crock-Pot on the "warm" setting to infuse your honey in about a day. The honey will work on its own. The herbs will work on their own. Studies tend to suggest that they work better together.

---

25 http://www.ncbi.nlm.nih.gov/pmc/articles/PMC3273858.
26 http://www.ncbi.nlm.nih.gov/pmc/articles/PMC3757282.
27 http://www.ncbi.nlm.nih.gov/pmc/articles/PMC3977104.
28 http://www.ncbi.nlm.nih.gov/pubmed/16379555.

When you find any boil of any size, even if it's small, assume it's MRSA and apply the herbal honey to the infected area and cover with gauze. Change out often by washing with a hot-to-tolerance (be careful not to burn the skin) wet cloth. If you do this as early as possible when the boil is still small, and support the immune system at the same time, you stand the best chance of preventing a much larger problem. If the boil is quite large, and it can grow to several inches in diameter in a very short time, you can still apply the honey before lancing and draining the boil. Putting a hot-to-tolerance towel on the boil will help draw it out. If there's a large space where the pus created a pocket, soak a strip of gauze in the herbal honey and pack the wound. You can also pour the honey into the wound and cover with a bandage.

Most of the time, draining the boil is all that's necessary. But sometimes the infection refuses to go away. If it persists, it can move deeper into the body and may require surgery to clean out the infected pus from a joint. It may even require amputation as a last-ditch effort to stop the spread and save the patient. There's only so much you can do for an MRSA infection at home. Draining a boil is one thing. Amputation is an entirely different situation. There's no good answer to this problem, other than preventative measures and swift response before the problem gets out of hand.

Tea tree and geranium essential oils are another option for topical care.[29] [30] Essential oils should be diluted in a carrier oil before applying directly to the skin. For MRSA, I would opt for a very light, non-pore-clogging oil, like grape seed oil or hemp seed oil. Hazelnut oil is actually quite drying, and as long as there are no nut allergies, would make an ideal choice.

Two final topical remedies are worthy of mention. The first is a commercial product called Alliderm Gel, which uses a patented process to keep allicin, a highly antimicrobial constituent from crushed or chopped garlic, stable. This seems like a useful product to keep in a first aid or trauma kit, as the allicin in garlic has a short half-life. That half-life is about six days, longer if preserved with a combination of alcohol

---

29 http://www.ncbi.nlm.nih.gov/pubmed/15066738.
30 http://www.ncbi.nlm.nih.gov/pubmed/15555788.

and water, such as in a tincture. Using an alcohol-based tincture on an open wound would sting, at the very least. Having this gel on hand would be very useful. You could also apply a fresh solution of crushed garlic in water or garlic honey to the infection.

The second and last remedy for topical infections comes from an unlikely source: an Anglo-Saxon herbal book written about one thousand years ago. A multidisciplinary group of scientists and researchers at the University of Nottingham found a remedy for an eye salve in *Bald's Leechbook* (doctors and healers were called "leeches" in reference to their frequent use of leeches in medicine) that was highly effective against MRSA. This medieval remedy demonstrated a level of sophistication not previously attributed to medicine of the period. It consisted of crushed garlic, crushed onion (or leek), wine, and bovine stomach bile.

The concoction was to be made in a brass vessel. The research team had to approximate without precise measurements for the garlic and onion, bile salts dissolved in water, and wine from a Glastonbury orchard, and used a piece of copper in the liquid instead of a brass vessel. Bile salts can be purchased in supplement stores or online and are sometimes labeled as bile acids. The resulting mixture proved highly active against MRSA.

For Airborne Transmission. MRSA and VISA can be sent into the air either through sneezing or coughing, or even through the act of making a bed. They can be catapulted in the air, off the bed linens, and sent through the air ducts, recirculating air throughout a building.

There are four ways I can see to mitigate this situation indoors.
• Negative pressure
• Aromatherapy
• Herbal smoke
• PPE (personal protective equipment)

Negative pressure is when you create a draft drawing the air out of the room, for example, by placing a fan pointing outward in a window.

Aromatherapy is the use of aromatic, volatile oils distilled from plants. These oils are most often called essential oils, which are highly antimicrobial. The oils I would select are thyme, geranium (*Pelargonium graveolens*), and peppermint.[31, 32, 33] To use essential oils to clean the air, you'll need an ionizing diffuser. Just follow the instructions on the diffuser.

Another reason to have an ionizing diffuser on hand is for respiratory infections. If faced with a respiratory MRSA infection, there really isn't going to be any way to know that it's MRSA without a lab test to confirm it. There are many essential oils that work wonders on respiratory infections from the common cold to influenza to pneumonia. A breathing treatment with essential oils and an ionizing diffuser, sometimes called a nebulizing diffuser, can address multiple problems with the same solution. Good choices would be thyme, juniper, peppermint, lavender, rosemary, eucalyptus (*Eucalyptus globulus*; use rosalina [*Melaleuca ericifolia*]) instead of eucalyptus in children under ten, or geranium. If using with children, thyme can be a harsh oil. Keep it to a minimum in your blend, or eliminate it. It's best to avoid using essential oils with very young children.

When I say, "herbal smoke," I'm referring to the art of burning herbs to fill a space with aromatic smoke. I'm not referring to the oral inhalation of tobacco or other herbs. Herbal smoke may seem strange if you haven't used it before. Many people associate burning herbs and resins with Catholic Church incense, with New Age stores, or perhaps with tribal and traditional healers. Herbal smoke, however, has documented benefits as an air purifier.[34] I generally make a bundle by binding lengths of herbs together with natural twine. The end can be lit, allowed to burn for a couple of minutes, and then extinguished. The ends of the herbs will still smolder and glow red. Plenty of smoke will result. The bundle of herbs I would pick for respiratory help include sage, thyme, lavender, mugwort (*Artemisia vulgaris*), and rosemary.

Personal protective equipment (PPE) is protective clothing and gear that you wear to prevent infection. Common PPE items would include protective gloves, face masks, face shields, smocks, hair nets, and booties. There are also complete fluid-proof suits with hood and

---

31 http://www.ncbi.nlm.nih.gov/pubmed/19576738.
32 http://www.ncbi.nlm.nih.gov/pubmed/19292822.
33 http://www.ncbi.nlm.nih.gov/pubmed/?term=peppermint+oil+mrsa.
34 http://www.ncbi.nlm.nih.gov/pubmed/17030480.

enclosed face shields with ventilated face masks, often worn with both vinyl gloves covered with rubber gloves, and rubber boots over Tyvek pants. At the other end of the spectrum, PPE can be improvised with heavy-duty contractor's trash bags, duct tape, and goggles.

For UTIs. Urinary tract infections (UTIs) are pure misery. MRSA is sometimes a culprit in recurring UTIs. MRSA does not always leave the body after an active infection is stopped. It may lie dormant in the body, waiting for another opportunity to emerge. Recurrent UTIs are a good example of this. Testing strips for UTI infections to confirm that the problem really is a UTI are available from Amazon.

The tincture I use in my practice is made from equal parts of bilberry, juniper berry, dandelion, corn silk, nettle seed, and *Phellodendron amurense,* or any berberine-containing herb, such as coptis (*Coptis chinensis*), yellowroot (*Xanthorhiza simplicissima*), barberry (Berberis vulgaris), or Oregon grape root (*Mahonia aquifolium*).

I tincture the herbs separately and then combine equal portions of them. You could also use equal portions of each herb in a mason jar and tincture the herbs all at once. It's really your preference. Allow to steep for six weeks, strain out all the plant material, blend together if necessary, bottle and label. The dosage is 30 to 60 drops three to six times per day.

For Septicemia. Unfortunately, sometimes MRSA makes it into the bloodstream. This is called septicemia. From the bloodstream, MRSA can travel throughout the body. Symptoms for septicemia are:

- Fever and difficulty maintaining body temperature
- Elevated pulse
- Decreased urination
- Intestinal discomforts

This is a life-threatening situation. You're no better off staying at home than you are going to a VISA- or VRSA-infected facility at this point. The kinds of antibiotics that would be administered are beyond what you could buy for fish.

If for some reason hospitals were no longer treating patients, if there are no longer antibiotics to treat this, and you simply have no other choice, I suggest trying the following for septicemia or sepsis, as well as if a skin infection of MRSA will not heal, or you suspect the infection has moved into the bones or joints.

The following suggestions are based originally on the recommendations in Stephen Harrod Buhner's book, *Herbal Antibiotics*, which I then adjusted for clients in my own herbal practice. These would be clients struggling with MRSA, and nothing that the doctors prescribed seemed to help. The remedy comes in two tinctures, one given every hour, the other every two hours.

First, make a tincture out of equal parts of the following herbs. You can tincture them separately or all in one jar; it's up to you. Steep for six weeks, strain, label, bottle, and administer 60 drops every two hours until the fever has broken.

- Sida (*Sida acuta*)
- Bidens (*Bidens pilosa*)
- Sweet Annie (*Artemisia annua*)
- Black pepper (*Piper nigrum*)

Next, make a second tincture out of the following herbs following the steps above. These are taken in greater quantity and more frequently. The dosage would be 60 drops, but this tincture is taken every hour. Do this in combination with the above tincture every two hours.

- Echinacea (*Echinacea angustfolia*)
- Red sage (*Salvia miltiorrhiza*)
- Dong quai (*Angelica sinensis*)

As I have shown, MRSA, VISA, and VRSA can be contracted in many ways, in many locations, and through many activities, and it can attack the body in multiple ways. It will challenge us to be prepared for anything. This is a tricky and adaptable bacteria that stands a good chance of being the next great pandemic.

CHAPTER 4

Threat Level II:
Coronaviruses, Viral Hemorrhagic Fever

Threat Level II diseases are similar to Threat Level I diseases. They are deadly, infectious diseases that are easily spread from person to person and have high mortality rates. But they scored slightly fewer threat assessment points. While both illnesses at this level are active pandemics right now, they are active thousands of miles away. There's good containment in place now for each, but that won't prevent an infected person who is asymptomatic from bringing one of these diseases to the United States. All air travel would have to stop to prevent that circumstance. One of these diseases has its epicenter in Saudi Arabia, which has extensive foreign business interests and daily flights in and out of the country, and that's highly unlikely to stop.

Coronaviruses (SARS, MERS)

THREAT ASSESSMENT POINTS	
THREAT	POINTS
Current Pandemic	3
Transmission: Moderate	2
Treatment: Lacking	3
Mortality Rate: 50% or lower	2
TOTAL POINTS	10

Coronaviruses are fairly common viruses, most of which do not cause illness in humans. Of those that do, they typically cause mild to moderate respiratory illness. Coronaviruses are so called because their surface is covered in spikes with a crown-like appearance. It has a sort of halo, or corona. Coronaviruses are enveloped, RNA viruses. This means that they have greater defenses and are more likely to mutate. While most coronaviruses present little to no risk to human health, some are capable of serious, even fatal outcomes.

A coronavirus infection appears much like influenza, sharing symptoms such as congestion, coughing, fever, headache, body aches, sore throat, and muscle pain. But you wouldn't be able to tell the difference between an influenza and a coronavirus infection based on observation of the symptoms alone. That requires a test. Like influenza, coronaviruses can lead to difficulty breathing, the necessity for oxygen, cytokine storms, and ultimately, respiratory failure. Severe coronavirus illness is also similar to influenza because it's more severe for those who are weakest: the elderly, those with compromised immune systems, and especially patients with preexisting chronic illnesses.

Two coronaviruses that have proven deadly are severe acute respiratory syndrome (SARS) and Middle East respiratory syndrome (MERS). The viruses are related, are both zoonotic illnesses, and produce similar respiratory symptoms. The animal origin of SARS is not known. Several potential animal hosts have been identified, including bats, birds, and even civets. Human infection of MERS is believed to have originated by close contact with infected camels. Both viruses are spread in much the same way as influenza, by contact and water droplets in the air. SARS broke out in China, the most populous nation on earth. While we're lucky that the disease was contained, it did kill over eight thousand people.

SARS. An outbreak of the novel coronavirus SARS in 2002–2003 put the world into a panic when this mysterious illness mutated to infect people. The outbreak began in China, spread to Singapore and Vietnam, and then traveled east to Toronto and San Francisco. By 2003 SARS had infected people in a total of thirty-seven nations.

Even if a patient did recover from the acute symptoms of SARS, that person would move into a chronic phase. This phase included conditions such as pulmonary fibrosis (scar tissue on the lungs causing ongoing shortness of breath), which is not unusual for a severe, respiratory infection. Another serious outcome of chronic SARS is the blood supply to the bones being cut off, either resulting in osteoporosis (bone becoming porous and weak) or necrosis (cell death). To date, there's no vaccine for SARS.

MERS. Then there's the more recent "cousin" of SARS, MERS. At the time of this writing, October 2015, MERS is active in a second wave of an outbreak that began in 2012. It has spread from Saudi Arabia to South Korea and Germany. While official reports in Western media cling to narratives that say the number of infected is declining, WHO has warned that the situation in South Korea is more complex than previously thought, and to expect more cases, with ongoing transmission in the community. This is despite over five thousand people currently under quarantine in South Korea.

When the outbreak began, the mortality rate of MERS was an almost unimaginable 60 percent. This rate is from a study from July 2013 that was published in the *Lancet*.[35] The study provides some crucial information for understanding which populations are most susceptible to this infection. Of this 60 percent, 96 percent had "underlying comorbid medical disorders." A whopping 68 percent of the 96 percent with chronic illnesses had diabetes, making diabetes the number one risk factor for a fatal outcome from MERS. Chronic renal disease was number two, with 49 percent.

While there are many similarities between SARS and MERS, this same study also showed a few major differences as well. MERS at the time of the study was somewhat less contagious than SARS,

---

35 http://www.thelancet.com/journals/laninf/article/PIIS1473-
3099%2813%2970204-4/abstract?rss=yes.

but progressed to respiratory failure five days sooner than seen in SARS.[36] Furthermore, SARS seemed to target the healthy, young adult population, unlike MERS, which seemed to target the weaker, older, and chronically ill population. But this recent outbreak of MERS in South Korea suggests that MERS may have mutated, as transmission is happening easily in both the hospital setting and in the community.

As tracking and reporting for MERS cases improved, more of the mild to moderate cases were reported, dropping the mortality rate down to 30 percent. But that mortality rate is nothing to sneeze at. It's higher than the influenza outbreak of 1918, and on par with some strains of Ebola. The current wave of this outbreak in South Korea is estimated at just over 12 percent, but with more cases expected, the actual mortality rate is unknown. On April 24, 2014, the United States had its first diagnosis of MERS. An American doctor working in the Middle East traveled from Saudi Arabia, which is the epicenter of the MERS outbreak, to London, and then to the United States by plane. He took a bus from the airport in Chicago to Indiana to attend a medical conference. On April 27, he began to feel ill, with shortness of breath, fever, and coughing. He was admitted as a patient on April 28 and cared for in an isolation unit.

This first MERS patient's movements were retraced, and the people who came in contact with him tested. Another conference attendee tested positive for MERS antibodies. The only contact between the two individuals was sitting at a conference table and shaking hands. Still, experts at the Centers for Disease Control insisted that close contact was necessary for transmission of MERS. A few days later, another patient arrived in Florida from Saudi Arabia who tested positive for active MERS. Quick response and treatment in an isolation unit prevented the further spread of the virus.[37]

---

36 http://www.ahcmedia.com/blogs/2-hicprevent/post/133687-mers-cov-case-series-a-60-mortality-rate-in-patients-with-complications-of-diabetes-hypertension-chronic-cardiac-and-renal-disease.

37 http://www.cdc.gov/coronavirus/mers/us.html.

Saudi Arabia is a hub of international business and travel. This made the likelihood of MERS spreading internationally not just a possibility but more of a matter of time. Not only is Saudi Arabia the MERS outbreak epicenter, it's also the destination of one to two million Muslim pilgrims to Mecca, known as the Hajj. Bringing that many people into the epicenter of the MERS outbreak who will then return home to all parts of the globe is a recipe for a pandemic.

In June 2014 a little over one hundred new previously unreported cases from Saudi Arabia were discovered through an audit of records. The Saudis maintain that they did not intentionally underreport MERS cases. Shortly after this, MERS faded from the news, as the media turned to focus on the Ebola crisis.

MERS hasn't gone away. It's spread to South Korea, where it has readily been transmitted person to person. This outbreak began on May 20, 2015, when a man from South Korea returned home from traveling in Saudi Arabia. Upon his return, he became ill and went to the hospital. Nine days later, he was diagnosed with MERS. From this one case, over 6,700 people were placed in isolation either in their homes or in medical facilities, schools were closed, and the South Korean economy has suffered greatly. So far, 154 people have tested positive for MERS, and 24 have died. It was the South Korean government's swift action that prevented a larger outbreak. At the same time, having thousands of people's lives disrupted for an imposed isolation comes with an economic cost that has yet to be calculated.

MERS is still active in Saudi Arabia. All it takes is one traveler who leaves Saudi Arabia without knowing he or she is ill for it to spread again. Will it come back to the United States? Will we respond swiftly enough to contain it if it comes? I hope so, because according to the CDC, one in every two adults in the United States has a chronic illness, such as diabetes, hypertension, chronic kidney disease, and so on. South Korea has about one in four adults with a chronic illness. The harsh reality is that one in two adults have a greater risk of dying if infected with MERS. A 50 percent mortality rate among adults is a reasonable expectation for a MERS outbreak in the United States.

Coronavirus Symptoms and Transmission

To be accurate, this section applies to those types of coronavirus capable of causing severe illness in humans, specifically SARS and MERS.

Coronavirus Risk Factors

- Travel to an area with an outbreak, such as Saudi Arabia, with MERS.
- Contact with a person who has been to a region with active coronavirus cases.
- Contact with camels, including their bodily fluids, unpasteurized camel milk, and camel meat. Preexisting condition, especially diabetes, cardiovascular disease, liver disease, or kidney disease.

Coronavirus Symptoms

Symptoms range from mild to severe. Some people never even know they're sick; others are facing a fatal illness and respiratory failure. Symptoms mimic that of influenza:

- Fever
- Body aches and pains
- Fatigue
- Coughing
- Congestion
- Sore throat
- Shortness of breath
- Diarrhea/intestinal discomfort

Symptoms can progress and lead to secondary infections, such as viral or bacterial pneumonia, or a lack of oxygen, causing:

- Dizziness
- Blue fingertips or lips
- Rapid heartbeat
- Respiratory failure

Coronavirus Transmission

Transmission of SARS and MERS is similar to influenza. It takes place through water droplets in the air, as well as close contact with an infected person. MERS is also passed from camel to person by drinking the milk or urine of an infected camel.

Coronavirus Response

Conventional Medical Response

Coronaviruses can be prevented in much the same way as other respiratory illnesses, like influenza and tuberculosis. Avoid crowded places, such as schools, movie theaters, shopping centers, and any place with poor ventilation.

Preventative measures, such as wearing face masks and gloves, are appropriate. If you're called on to care for a person with MERS, then a gown would be a smart thing to have. Create negative pressure using a window fan pointing outward, and make sure to section off the room from the healthy people in the home.

There's no antiviral medication for MERS at this time. Conventional care for mild cases focuses on symptom relief, much like the flu. A patient with a severe coronavirus infection is really a case for a hospital, but if the hospital reaches surge capacity for this or any other calamity, there wouldn't be a hospital available. Hospital treatments are oxygen therapy, perhaps intubation and suctioning to keep airways open, along with antibiotics for secondary bacterial infections. While there are emergency first aid oxygen kits on the market, this is appropriate only if there's no alternative and no doctor or hospital available.

Natural and Herbal Response

As an herbalist, I would look to herbal steams, aromatherapy treatments with essential oils, and antimicrobial herbal formulas for effective, alternative treatment and disinfectant options. Here are those that make the top of my list for coronaviruses.

Herbal Steams. Warm a pot of water to steaming, and remove from heat. Being careful, as steam can burn, add any of the following herbs to the pot, and inhale the humidity and aromatics for as long as you're comfortable:

- Thyme
- Juniper
- Rosemary
- Sage
- Red pepper flakes
- Lavender
- Peppermint

Respiratory Infection Tea. This tea is from my book, *Prepper's Natural Medicine*. It works wonders to make coughing more productive and comfortable. Mix a large batch of the following dried herbs and make ahead of time. Use 1 teaspoon of the mixture to steep your tea for about fifteen minutes and drink four to six cups daily to help calm symptoms.

- 2 cups hyssop flowers
- 1½ cups mullein (*Verbascum thapsus*) leaves
- 1½ cups slippery elm (*Ulmus fulva*) bark
- 1 cup elecampane root
- ½ cup coltsfoot aerial parts
- ½ cup marshmallow root
- ½ cup spearmint (*Mentha spicata*) leaves
- ½ cup whole cloves
- ½ cup licorice root
- ½ cup thyme leaves

Coronavirus Tincture. While I wish I could say, "Here's a tincture with a blend of herbs effective against coronaviruses," I cannot. The United States has seen only a few hundred SARS cases, with even less confirmed to be SARS, and this was over a decade ago. I can count on one hand how many MERS patients have been treated in the United States. The opportunity to study the effect of herbs on MERS patients hasn't been available. But I can say that based on what I know of these herbs, I believe that the following blend would be helpful. Feel free to adapt this as you see fit.

Make tinctures of the following herbs, and then blend equal amounts of the finished tinctures into one container. I would administer 60 drops every two hours on the first day. If there were improvement, I would back it down to every three hours on the second day, and every four on the next day, and so on, as long as there is progress. If no improvement, I would keep it the same and wait another day. If it became more severe, I would increase the dose to every hour for one day and reassess.

- Japanese knotweed (*Fallopia japonica*)
- Elderflower
- Rhodiola
- Cordyceps (*Cordyceps sinensis*, a parasitic mushroom)
- Chinese skullcap
- Astragalus
- Red sage (*Salvia miltiorrhiza*)
- Thyme
- Bidens (*Bidens pilosa*)

Viral Hemorrhagic Fevers (VHFs): Ebola, Marburg, Lassa

THREAT ASSESSMENT POINTS	
THREAT	**POINTS**
Past Pandemic	1
Current Pandemic	3
Transmission: Moderate	2
Treatment: Lacking	3
TOTAL POINTS	9

Viral hemorrhagic fevers (VHFs) are groups of viruses that cause severe illness in multiple systems of the body, and in particular, the vascular system. The vascular system is responsible for circulating fluids, such as blood and lymph, throughout the body. When the vascular system cannot regulate itself, we see the hallmark hemorrhaging for which these viruses are known. The most well-known of these viruses is the Ebola virus.

These are uniquely dangerous viruses and are classified as biosafety level four (BSL-4) pathogens. At the start of the current Ebola outbreak, there were only four hospitals in the United States capable of treating patients with diseases caused by BSL-4 pathogens. These were:

- NIH Clinical Center in Bethesda, Maryland
- St. Patrick Hospital in Missoula, Montana
- Emory University Hospital in Atlanta, Georgia
- Nebraska Medical Center in Omaha, Nebraska

Between these four hospitals they had eleven beds. From October 2014 to February 2015, the number of hospitals capable of treating patients with Ebola or other VHF increased to fifty-five. But these newer facilities are all clustered around the original four hospitals, and there are eight of these hospitals in California alone. There's not an equipped hospital for every state in the United States.

While Ebola is the most commonly known hemorrhagic viral fever disease because of its exceedingly high mortality rate and its recent outbreak in West Africa, it's only one of many viruses that cause hemorrhagic fevers. There are four virus families that cause viral hemorrhagic fevers: arenaviruses, bunyaviruses, filoviruses, and flaviviruses.

Arenaviruses. Arenaviruses are zoonotic VHFs transmitted by rodents to people. This normally takes place when someone eats something contaminated by rodents, or if a person with a skin cut or break comes in contact with contaminated rodent excrement. There are a few that can be transmitted directly from person to person when coming in contact with their body fluids. These include Lassa virus, Machupo virus, and Lujo virus.

Lassa and Lujo both come from Africa. Lassa is endemic to the same region coping with the ongoing Ebola virus. Lujo is from South Africa, more specifically Zambia. Machupo, on the other hand, is found in South America, deep in the jungles of Bolivia.

Conventional wisdom has been that these are viruses of the deep, dark jungle and are not likely threats. But this is one lesson of the current Ebola outbreak: they can, and do, escape the jungle.

And while we're on the verge of a vaccine for Ebola, we saw several patients come to the United States and Canada with Ebola-like symptoms who turned out to have Lassa fever. While not Ebola, one could think of Lassa as Ebola's less deadly cousin. Lassa fever can result in up to 20 percent of patients requiring hospitalization, which would put a significant strain on our medical and economic systems, but carries only a 1 percent mortality rate. Still, it's not something you want to have to endure, and it can still kill. Person-to-person transmission is also less of a concern, as it's generally transmitted by rodents. That still doesn't preclude it from traveling. Plague also traveled by rodents.

Bunyaviruses. There are over three hundred viruses in this family. Bunyaviruses are not spread person to person but are transmitted by ticks, mosquitoes, fleas, and rodents. Occasionally, they can be transmitted by larger animals, including sheep. They can cause mild to severe illness, but thankfully, most are mild. There are some notable exceptions, though, including Crimean-Congo hemorrhagic fever (CCHF), Rift Valley fever virus (RVF), and hemorrhagic fever with renal syndrome (HFRS).

CCHF is found over a wide area of the globe, including eastern and southern Europe, the Mediterranean, the Middle East, India, Central Asia, and northwestern China. The virus that causes it is often found in agricultural production centers, slaughter facilities, and outdoors where CCHF is endemic. Treatment is largely supportive and has a mortality rate that can range from 9 percent to 50 percent.

RVF is found in eastern and southern Africa, and is transmitted to people through livestock. The people most at risk of RVF are the same as those at risk for CCHF: those working in agriculture, handling livestock, and working outdoors where RVF is endemic. Treatment is mostly supportive and has a mortality rate that varies between 1 percent and 15 percent depending on the strain.

HFRS is found almost all over the world and is caused by the Hantaan, Dobrava, Saaremaa, Seoul, and Puumala viruses. In the United States and Canada, however, our hantavirus strains cause hantavirus pulmonary syndrome. Hantavirus pulmonary syndrome is not a hemorrhagic viral fever disease, but I address it in Chapter 6, The Watch List. HFRS, however, is a viral hemorrhagic fever. Again, supportive care is provided, and there's a 5 percent to 15 percent mortality rate for HFRS patients.

Filoviruses. There are only three members of the Filoviridae virus family, and only two have made humans sick. The first is Marburgvirus, which was discovered in the 1960s in the German cities of Marburg and Frankfurt. Researchers there had been exposed to the tissues of infected monkeys. The second, and the one that made headlines for almost the entire year of 2014, is Ebolavirus.

If Lassa is Ebola's less deadly cousin, then Marburg is Ebola's equally deadly but rarely seen twin. It's found in more southern regions of Africa, but spreads in the exact same way as Ebola. And while it makes only a rare appearance, as recently as 2008, two separate travelers, one from the Netherlands and the other from the United States, both became ill with Marburg once they returned home, after visiting caves known to be home to the Marburg reservoir host, the African fruit bat.

First found in 1976 in the dark jungles of Zaire, now known as the Democratic Republic of the Congo, Ebolavirus was named for the river Ebola, and is often just referred to as Ebola. There are five species of the genus Ebolavirus, but only four that result in human illness. These are Bundibugyo virus, Sudan virus, Taï Forest virus (formerly Ivory Coast virus), and Ebola Zaire. The last one has been the most feared, with the highest mortality rate of 90 percent. Ebola Zaire has also been responsible for the most outbreaks and is cited as the virus responsible for the current Ebola outbreak in West Africa. The fifth type of Ebolavirus is Reston virus and has so far caused illness only in nonhuman primates.

The third type of Filoviridae is called Cuevavirus and is found in France, Spain, and Portugal. It has been found in bats native to the regions and is related to the Marburg and Ebola viruses. There has never been anyone known to have become ill from contact with the bats. Considering that one way people in Africa become infected with Ebolavirus is to eat bats, and people in France, Spain, and Portugal do not eat bats, perhaps this is why humans have not become sick with Cuevavirus.

Flaviviruses. Several flaviviruses cause illness, but a few specifically cause hemorrhagic viral fevers. Dengue from all over the tropics is spread by mosquitoes, Alkhurma is from Saudi Arabia and spread by ticks, and Omsk comes from Russia and is transmitted by either rodent or tick.

These different viruses all cause viral hemorrhagic fevers and share several commonalities.

- These viruses favor dark, tropical jungles.
- These are zoonotic diseases. They all share the same symptoms, progressing from minor to severe.
- Treatments are generally similar, largely centered on supportive care.

There are no approved vaccines for VHFs, though WHO recently announced that an Ebola vaccine may be approved very soon.[38] Let's hope that this comes to pass, as the promise of a vaccine is long overdue. A few viruses are treated with an antiviral medication called Ribavirin. There are several experimental drugs, though none have come to market. Most treatment is supportive, including administration of IV fluids, oxygen, dialysis, and supporting the body as problems come up in an effort to keep patients alive long enough to let their immune systems fight off the virus. None of these diseases has ever resulted in a global pandemic because they have traditionally favored particular regions: dark, dense, tropical forests. These are jungle diseases found both in the East and in the West. But the Ebola outbreak in West Africa hasn't been deterred, despite not being in a dark, dense jungle. Ebola has found its footing in both remote villages and the inner-city slums, and is both an urban and a rural issue now.

Given that Ebola is only one of many similar viruses and that all viruses have the ability to adapt, how long will it be before another VHF takes hold in an urban area, perhaps New Orleans or Miami, because a tick or mosquito was a hidden traveler on a plane and goes on to spread the virus to the mosquito population here? Something like that has already happened with another flavivirus, West Nile virus.

Viral Hemorrhagic Fever Symptoms and Transmission

VHF Risk Factors
- Travel to Africa, specifically to an area where there's an outbreak or where there has ever been an outbreak.
- Care for VHF patients or involved in the decontamination process of health care workers as they remove their PPEs.
- Conduct animal research.
- Eat undercooked "bushmeat," specifically bats, but also potentially, monkeys.

---

38 http://www.who.int/mediacentre/news/releases/2015/effective-ebola-vaccine/en.

- Come in contact with an infected person or the body of someone who died from a VHF.
- Participate in traditional funeral rituals from Africa involving the handling of a body of someone who died from a VHF.
- Prepare bodies for burial.

VHF Symptoms

As stated above, these viruses share many of the same symptoms. These include:

- Fever
- Aches and pains
- Flu-like symptoms
- Vomiting
- Diarrhea
- Dehydration
- Decreased ability to make blood clots, causing hemorrhaging
- Sudden decreases in blood pressure
- Renal failure
- Sepsis
- Multiple organ failure
- Death

VHF Transmission

Transmission may be from animal to person or directly from person to person. The primary animal vectors are bats, mice, rats, mosquitoes, ticks, and fleas. With the exception of the bunyaviruses, once in the human population, transmission takes place readily through bodily fluids.

Viral Hemorrhagic Fever Response

As mentioned above, the standard treatment for viral hemorrhagic fevers is supportive care. If there's an outbreak, the absolute best place for a patient is in a well-staffed, modern medical facility where fluids, vitals, and internal infections and organs can be best monitored and supported. It's a nice theory, but there's a huge flaw. If you recall the lessons learned in the first chapter, you know that such hospital care will not be available to all. If there were to be an outbreak of a VHF, we have already seen what can happen when medical facilities are overwhelmed, as they were and still are in West Africa, and are unprepared, as they were in Dallas with Thomas Eric Duncan. While we now have fifty-five hospitals capable of caring for a BSL-4 pathogenic disease, that's still going to leave most of the country without such a hospital. Local hospitals will have to scramble to put policies in place for how to deal with such an outbreak and will quickly reach surge capacity. Waiting rooms will fill with no help coming.

The biggest threat with hospitals not operating as normal may not be contracting a VHF. It might be a heart attack, it might be an infection from a cut, or it could be a worsening of one's diabetes, and so on. You must be prepared to deal with common injuries and illnesses on your own. Improving your health ahead of time will improve your chances of not having a major illness during a time when hospitals may not be able to see you.

And if, just if, you're forced into the situation of caring for family or other people in your group, when someone ultimately comes down with a viral hemorrhagic fever, all is not lost. There have been heroic stories of survival from West Africa during this outbreak. One woman took care of her entire family protected by nothing but improvised PPE out of trash bags and duct tape.[39] She kept them hydrated and clean until they were able to fight off the infection. Three out of four of her family members survived.

Conventional Medical Response

Fluids and keeping the patients hydrated has proven to be the number one most important step in treating Ebola patients. It's also one of the most problematic. The best way is to get the patient to drink plenty of fluids with oral rehydration salts to maintain electrolyte balance. This won't be easy, as many patients may be in so much pain they may not want to drink anything. They must. Otherwise, they risk a sudden drop in blood pressure, shock, and death.

If they won't drink, there are only two other options. Both have their pros and cons. The first is to start administration of IV fluids. This will require you to learn how to start an IV, make your own sterile saline to store at home, and stock up on IV supplies. Intravenous fluids are the

---

39 http://www.cnn.com/2014/09/25/health/ebola-fatu-family/

gold standard for hydration. But if the person is hemorrhaging, this may not be possible. The puncture may cause too much bleeding to start an IV line.

The final option is to use proctoclysis, also known as a Murphy Drip. An enema bag is used to create a slow drip into the rectum. If you've ever wondered what method was used in hospitals prior to administered fluids with an IV drip, this was it. Murphy Drips were used historically to help treat viral hemorrhagic fevers. The drawback is that while normally anything inserted into the anus is readily absorbed, which is why many medications are administered via suppositories, it's not ideal. Because of the severe diarrhea, the body is not able to function normally. Not all the fluid would be absorbed as well as it should. On the other hand, this method is far easier to learn at home than learning how to start an IV. If you can get the training to start an IV, get it. If not, then this method is an acceptable, if not ideal, alternative.

Natural and Herbal Response

There are no approved medicines for Ebola, which has led to many questions to the herbalist community wondering if we have anything that might work. The short answer is no. Let's hope that the vaccine being tested on the Ebola virus will be fast-tracked for approval. What normally happens during an Ebola outbreak is that the virus rips through a village so fast that there's no time to test anything, pharmaceutical or herbal. Besides that, because of how infectious and dangerous the disease is, and the resulting security measures around treatment facilities, no herbalist is going to get close enough to an Ebola patient to ever test anything.

There has never been any in vivo (in a live patient) testing of natural remedies of any type against Ebola. So claims of natural remedies for Ebola, which unfortunately have been made during this crisis by sales representatives of two multi-level-marketing essential oil companies, are horribly misleading at best, and preying on people's fears for profit at worst.

Any strategy an herbalist might come up with for any VHF is pure conjecture. It might work, it might not. It would be a theory, an educated guess. And there wouldn't be an opportunity to find out if it worked, unless there were such a calamity as a global viral hemorrhagic fever pandemic at your doorstep.

This is something I thought about a lot over the past year and a half since this outbreak began, and largely because of the e-mails I received from my blog's readers. So, if I were faced with such a nightmarish hypothetical situation, and I were forced to come up with some type of treatment plan, where would I start?

I would start by looking at conventional treatment, and include plenty of oral rehydration salts in the supplies. Be prepared to administer fluids via an IV or via a Murphy Drip, depending on your skill set. Next, I would first look at the symptoms being presented and try to provide palliative care. The symptoms are usually initial flu-like symptoms, nausea and vomiting, severe diarrhea, hemorrhage, dehydration, sudden drop in blood pressure, shock, and then organ failure.

Flu-Like Symptoms. I would look to those herbs that help with flu symptoms, so I might try a decoction of ginger, cloves, and garlic with honey for those very first days where VHFs mimic flu symptoms. It may provide some comfort for the general aches, sore throat pain, and malaise. Chicken broth is also comforting to flu-like symptoms and will help hydrate the individual. Because of the vomiting and intense diarrhea, the patient may as well go in fully hydrated.

I would also consider including herbs such as elderberry and boneset. Both support the immune system: elderberry is considered an antiviral herb for the flu, and boneset (*Eupatorium perfoliatum*) may help keep that fever at bay. It opens the body up and allows the sweat to pour out. Sweat is one of the few ways the body detoxifies itself and a far better way to cool down a fever than artificially forcing it to be lower.

Nausea, Vomiting, and Diarrhea. For the nausea and vomiting, I might try more ginger, or perhaps peppermint, or chamomile. I would also sweeten with honey, as individuals who are nauseated and vomiting could do with a bit of sugar to get that awful taste out of their mouths. For the diarrhea, I might try a decoction of something astringent, such as oak bark. The hope would be to slow down the vomiting and diarrhea, providing a chance for the patient to rehydrate by sipping on oral rehydration salts.

Hemorrhage. Severe hemorrhaging, especially out of the mouth, nose, and eyes, is the image most people have of hemorrhagic fevers. That's why this group of viruses is known as viral hemorrhagic fevers. This dramatic symptom, however, is actually more the exception than the rule.

Hemorrhaging happens in the day or two before death. The liver has been infected and can't produce the proteins necessary to form blood clots. At the same time, the immune system has gone into overdrive, releasing cytokines and causing body-wide inflammation. This inflammation causes weakened blood vessels to burst. The body forms clots all over until the proteins necessary for forming blood clots are completely used up. If the liver has been infected and compromised, it cannot make enough blood-clotting factor, and hemorrhaging begins. I would begin administering liver-protective and supportive herbs like milk thistle (*Silybum marianum*) and burdock (*Arctium lappa*) immediately if a VHF is suspected.

To help increase clotting, yarrow (*Achillea millefolium*) and shepherd's purse (*Capsella bursa-pastoris*) may be helpful. These are both used to stop bleeding, mostly with external wounds. They have also been used for internal bleeding, such as uterine hemorrhage during labor.

Another cause for hemorrhage with VHF is that the virus sometimes causes intense inflammation in the blood vessels and breaks down their inner walls. It weakens these walls, and eventually fluid migrates out. Herbs such as bilberry (*Vaccinium myrtillus*), horse chestnut (*Aesculus hippocastanum*) seeds, and butcher's broom (*Ruscus aculeatus*) are known for strengthening blood vessels. At the same time, I would likely include turmeric and yerba mansa (*Anemopsis californica*), as I have had the most success with reducing inflammation with these herbs.

Dehydration, Sudden Drop in Blood Pressure, and Shock. Vomiting and diarrhea can easily lead to dehydration. This, combined with hemorrhaging blood vessels, can lead to sudden drops in blood pressure, shock, and then death. It's imperative to keep the patient sipping fluids with oral rehydration salts. These can be purchased and stored for later use. That's more convenient than making them yourself, but you can do so by mixing 2 tablespoons of sugar or honey with ½ teaspoon of sea salt in 1 quart of water.

Regular table salt will not provide all the minerals that sea salt provides, because they're removed from table salt during processing. You could also use coconut water in place of regular water. Boxes of coconut water are available by the case at better wholesale clubs, store reasonably well, and already contain electrolytes, making coconut water a great option for rehydration.

Organ Failure. VHFs, like Ebola and Marburg, can lead to the failure of multiple organs. This is most likely going to be beyond the skill sets of most people preparing for such events. If hospital care is at all available, use it!

You'll likely not have a dialysis machine. If nothing else, have some nettle (*Urtica dioica*) seed tincture on hand for renal complications. Again, it's certainly not a guarantee, but nettle seed tincture has some encouraging, if limited, documented success associated with treating kidney failure. Then again, with VHFs, nothing is guaranteed, and I would rather have one more option to exhaust than not try anything.

Hawthorn (*Crataegus monogyna*) is the herb most associated with supporting the heart. But if the patient does have a heart attack, you would really need to have a portable defibrillator. These are expensive, but can be purchased online for between $1,000 and $2,000. This is far more accessible than something like a dialysis machine for the kidneys and an absolute necessity for anyone concerned about heart attacks.

A pulse oximeter, blood pressure cuff, and a stethoscope are necessary to monitor the amount of oxygen in the blood, as well as to record blood pressure. But heart attack is only one way the heart may suffer. Heart failure may require surgery, and unless you're a trained surgeon with an operating room at home, this is one of those unfortunate times when there really is nothing more one can do.

Putting This All Together

It's important to demonstrate how one might go about putting even a theoretical protocol for a disease together, even if there's no opportunity to test it. This is how one would approach not only a disease from far away but also emerging diseases for which we have no natural immunity against and no established treatments.

So what would this hypothetical treatment look like?

- A tincture formula containing elderberry, boneset, turmeric, and yerba mansa for flu-like symptoms, fever, and inflammation. Start immediately and continue throughout the treatment.
- Decoction of garlic, ginger, clove, and cinnamon with honey to sooth initial flu-like symptoms. Take as needed.
- Chicken broth for comfort from flu-like symptoms and later for rehydration, and oral rehydration salts for rehydration. Start immediately and continue throughout the treatment.
- A tincture formula containing milk thistle, burdock, hawthorn berry, bilberry, horse chestnut seeds, and butcher's broom, to protect the liver, heart, and blood vessels. Start immediately and continue throughout the treatment.
- A tincture of nettle seeds in case of kidney failure.
- A tincture of either yarrow or shepherd's purse to encourage blood clotting. Take as needed.

While the above might provide some comfort until the body fights off the illness, the best strategy is to not get sick in the first place. Have the knowledge and means to go into SIRQ and do what you can to avoid contact with other people or with animal vectors. If ever in the presence of someone with a VHF, your PPE must completely cover you, and you'll need help to remove your PPE safely.

VHFs are definitely the nightmare scenario. Thankfully, there seems to be progress toward a vaccine. Assuming the vaccine works, and it becomes readily available, not just available to a privileged class, this may shift Ebola and Ebola-like diseases farther down my threat level point system. However, since I don't count my chickens before they hatch, it remains, for now, at Threat Level II.

CHAPTER 5

Threat Level III:
Terrorism / Human Error (Smallpox, Plague), the Surprise

Threat Level III has two threats that pose unique challenges that the other levels do not. This threat level brings in human involvement and the unknown. These two variables make for unstable, unpredictable, and potentially devastating tragedies. At the same time, the two diseases considered for the human factor, regardless of whether the human involvement was intentional or accidental, are not easy to access. The unknown category deals with diseases we have yet to even imagine. We would have no natural immune response. No known defense. There would be no medication known to cure it. But there's no way to know when the next unknown disease will make itself known.

The Human Factor
(Smallpox, Plague)

THREAT ASSESSMENT POINTS	
THREAT	**POINTS**
Past Pandemic	1
Transmission: Moderate	2
Treatment: Difficult	2
Mortality Rate: Unknown	2
TOTAL POINTS	7

Human actions are not always accurate or benevolent. The human factor we need to be aware of for pandemic preparedness is the release of a deadly pathogen into the environment, through either human error or bioterrorism.

Just as the viral hemorrhagic fevers in the previous section are considered BSL-4 pathogens, there are laboratories in the United States, Russia, and around the globe that handle microorganisms at this same level. The publicly stated purpose of such labs and the storage and study of such microorganisms is for our protection. In case there were ever an outbreak of these diseases in the future, we would have a sample on hand to develop a vaccine or other medication as soon as possible, rather than start from scratch. The National Institutes of Health has ranked such pathogens into categories A, B, and C, with A being the most virulent and dangerous.

Human Error. Just the fact that these laboratories and their samples of deadly viruses and bacteria even exist places us all at risk from either bioterrorism or simple human error. Just last year in July 2014, an unsecured box was found in a storage closet at the National Institutes of Health. The vials in the box contained smallpox. They were made in 1954 but were supposed to have been sent to the FDA in 1972. No one knows how they ended up in the closet or why their whereabouts were never questioned. The vials were sent to CDC for testing, and two were determined to contain viable smallpox virus.

We're all very lucky that no one accidentally dropped or damaged the improperly stored box or, even worse, stole it. Smallpox is a contagious, deadly virus that causes fever and puss-filled "pox" all over the skin and internal organs. Victims die by drowning in their own fluids. CDC, the very folks we depend on for information on infectious diseases, has made major errors of its own. CDC has accidentally mailed pathogenic microorganisms at least five times in the past decade. These pathogens include avian influenza, anthrax, and botulism.

Another accidental release of a BSL-4 pathogen was in the former Soviet Union city of Sverdlovsk. The military base in the city accidentally released anthrax into the civilian population in 1979. During a shift change, a clogged chimney was removed for cleaning, but not replaced before the next shift came on duty.[40] There was a short period where anthrax belched out the open chimney in a cone-shaped plume across the city and into the countryside for several miles.

Initially, the government attempted to cover up the incident by blaming the anthrax on bad meat. That was not believable for two reasons. First, if it had been from contaminated meat and not a plume, then those infected would have come from all over the city. Instead, they came from only within the path of the cone. Second, there wasn't that much meat in the local population's diet to begin with. There was great pressure to keep the production of inhalation anthrax secret, since the Soviet Union had agreed to the terms set down at the Biological Weapons Convention in 1972, agreeing to discontinue the use and production of all biological weapons.

Bioterrorism. In the age of the never-ending War on Terror, one of the most frightening forms of terror is the bioterrorism attack. The intentional release of a deadly pathogen may not be detected for days or even weeks, and may also appear as a naturally occurring phenomenon. For example, if a particularly virulent influenza strain were to be

---

40 *Medicine Science and Dreams: The Making of Physician-Scientists*, by David A. Schwartz (Springer, 2011).

released in the middle of winter in a major city, such as Chicago or New York, would anyone think that it had been intentionally released?

The worst bioterrorism attack in the United States happened in 1984 in Dallas, Oregon. A religious cult called the Rajneeshees fled from India and acquired a 64,000-acre property in the Oregon town. In their desire to expand their borders, the cult encroached into neighboring towns, attempting to rename them. They wore red clothing, the highest-ranking woman was called "queen," and the cult had its own security team. The Rajneeshees and the locals had a tense, uncooperative relationship. The county denied the cult the permits required to build a city on property it had bought.

The cult's strategy was to flood the county government with cult members in an attempt to get the building permits. The cult attempted to import by bus hundreds of homeless people to vote, but they were not allowed to vote. The cult's plan B was far more sinister. Cult members contaminated ten salad bars in the area with salmonella. A contaminated, brown fluid was hastily added to the salsa and salad dressing. The idea was to make so many people sick that they would stay home from the voting polls. This bioterror attack resulted in 751 people sickened and 45 hospitalized. The plot didn't work, and the cult's candidates lost. Locals always suspected the cult was behind the contaminated salad bars, but they couldn't prove it. The cult began to break down, and its members and leaders fled to other parts of the world. Upon searching the deserted compound, authorities found a full-scale bioterror laboratory.

More recently, concern over bioterrorism peaked when a laptop was recovered from an ISIS hideout in Syria. The laptop's owner had been teaching himself about bioterrorism and was planning an attack using the plague spread by rodents. Also of concern was the potential for terrorists to obtain a sample of Ebolavirus. When Ebola clinics were attacked and raided in Guinea and Liberia, all sorts of contaminated materials were stolen. Instead of a suicide bomber, a terrorist could be infected with Ebola immediately before getting on a plane heading anywhere in the world long before symptoms began to show.

Category A: Priority Pathogens. The National Institute for Allergies and Infectious Diseases has a list of infectious agents called "priority pathogens," organized by category. Category A priority pathogens are the most worrisome. For this book, I'm looking at only those illnesses that are both Category A pathogens and also transmitted person to person. Some, such as anthrax and botulism, are extremely dangerous and could take out large numbers of people in a short time. They would make an effective and deadly weapon. But the outbreak would go only as far as that weapon's range. Or, if an accidental release, only as far as the accidental spread would permit. In the case of plague, influenza, or smallpox, the likelihood of the disease turning into a pandemic is much greater because of the person-to-person transmission.

The Category A priority pathogens are transmitted person to person and are plague, smallpox, and certain VHFs, such as Ebola.[41] VHFs have already been discussed in detail, so I'll say only a few words here and move on to smallpox and plague.

We have seen that Ebola can come to the United States, and we have seen it transmitted in a hospital setting. We have seen Ebola patients survive in home settings with meager supplies, and we have seen Ebola patients survive in a hospital setting. Still, it carries with it a high mortality rate, and the illness itself is brutal even if the patient survives. We have seen that it doesn't take gaining access to a high-security laboratory to gain access to the virus, when raiding an Ebola clinic is far easier. We have now seen Ebola thrive in dark, dense jungle as well as in urban environments. But would an outbreak of Ebola or any other VHF take off in the United States? It would depend on a number of factors. How fast would our government's response be? As we saw in Nigeria, government security and screening measures, monitoring who came in and went out, nipped the Ebola outbreak in the bud before it could gain a foothold.

We have seen what human error did with bringing and spreading Ebola in Dallas with the Duncan case. As far as bioterror, it would most easily come in by multiple infected individuals at the same time,

---

41 http://www.niaid.nih.gov/topics/biodefenserelated/biodefense/pages/cata.aspx.

overwhelming our medical system. But according to Dr. William C. Patrick III in an interview on the PBS series *NOVA*,[42] in the former Soviet Union, bioterrorism scientists were able to weaponize Marburg, a virus similar to Ebola. Dr. Patrick spent three decades at Ft. Detrick, Maryland, specializing in germ warfare.

This raises the possibility of this technology being sold to terrorist organizations, as well as vulnerability of a bioweapon being used by the Russian government. The likelihood of a war with Russia would have seemed silly to many just a few years ago. But the political landscape is always changing, and disputes in Ukraine have brought out old rivalries. The potential of a VHF being used as a weapon remains a possibility.

Smallpox (*Variola major*) Overview

Risk Factors
- Not having been vaccinated
- Being exposed, easy to become infected

Smallpox is a viral infection most modern doctors have never seen. Smallpox was eradicated through an aggressive vaccination program. Vials of it still exist in what we hope are secure laboratories around the world. Smallpox presents with an extensive rash and high fever. There are four types, with *Variola major* being the most common, responsible for 90 percent of all infections. *Variola major* has a mortality rate of 30 percent, which puts it in the same lethality ballpark as MERS, and well above the mortality rate of the 1918 flu pandemic. The other types of smallpox, flat and hemorrhagic, are both rare, but usually fatal. *Variola minor*, the last type, is rarely fatal.

Symptoms
There's an incubation period for seven to seventeen days, with an average of twelve to fourteen days before symptoms begin. During this time, the patient is not contagious. The initial symptoms are flu-like, aches and pains, fatigue, and fever. Sometimes, there's nausea and

---

42 http://www.pbs.org/wgbh/nova/bioterror/biow_patrick.html.

vomiting. This lasts about two to four days, at which time the rash begins in the mouth. This is when smallpox is the most contagious, and the greatest care to not infect others must be taken.

After the sores from the rash break open in the mouth, the rash will become apparent on the skin. After three days, the rash will turn into bumps. Within twenty-four hours, these bumps will fill with fluid, and some will have a depression in the center similar to a belly button. This is useful to know in case an outbreak happens postdisaster and there are no hospitals or diagnostics available. At this point, the fever will spike again and remain high for the next four days while the bumps scab over. After this, the bumps will harden and form a crust, and eventually will fall off. The patient is contagious until all the bumps have fallen off, which should be approximately three weeks after the rash first formed on the skin. This often leaves the patient with massive scarring and pitting of the skin.

Meanwhile, this same rash is also forming on the body's inner tissues, only these do not get dry and crusty, by virtue of being inside the body. When this happens in the lungs and is severe, a person can drown in the fluid from the bumps when they burst.

Transmission
Smallpox is spread by face-to-face contact, through airborne water droplets. If you have smallpox, anyone with whom you share a close space, especially family members who may kiss, such as a parent cuddling a small child, are at risk.

Conventional Medical Response
We simply do not see naturally occurring infections of smallpox anymore. While there is a smallpox vaccine, it's no longer routinely given. Anyone under forty years old is unlikely to have received it. It's also unlikely that our government could supply us with enough vaccine in case of a bioterror attack or an accidental release.

Bottom line: there would likely be no available response from our modern medical system.

Natural and Herbal Response

While I know of no herbs effective at treating smallpox, there are two options for a natural response: either avoidance through SIRQ or a medieval form of inoculation called variolation. Lady Mary Wortley Montagu was the wife of a British ambassador. She brought the practice of variolation back with her to Britain in the early 1700s. A cut was made in a person's skin, and some of the dried scab made into a powder or some of the fluid from a scab was put into the cut. This resulted in a mortality rate of 1 percent to 2 percent, down from 30 percent, which was a massive improvement. But this practice was not foolproof: nothing in medicine ever is. The drawbacks were that the person might become infected, and there was a small chance of death. It also meant that there was a chance of spreading the smallpox further.

Smallpox is so virulent, so painful, and so deadly, and we are so ill-equipped to handle an outbreak of it, that variolation may be a viable way to respond to a medical system that would no doubt be overwhelmed. If you happen to be one of the very first to become sick with smallpox, you may be fortunate enough to get proper medical care.

Plague (*Yersinia Pestis*) Overview

Plague is well-known for killing millions of people in medieval Europe. It's a bacterial disease most often transmitted by infected fleas. Once the rodent being bitten by fleas dies, the fleas are highly active and looking for a new host. Dogs and cats may bring the fleas home, but cats are generally helpers in plague outbreaks, because they help reduce the rodent population. Flea bites, as well as contact with infected bodily fluids, result in bubonic plague. This is the most common form of plague infection.

Plague occurs naturally all over the world. We see a handful of cases every year in the western and southwestern regions of the United States, usually spring through fall. The spread of plague, however, has been managed with fast response by both medical teams and spraying of pesticides locally, but also because the parts of our country that have more plague cases tend to be rural and less populated. According to John

D. Clements, who heads the molecular pathogenesis and immunology program at Tulane University School of Medicine, weaponizing plague would be challenging. In an interview with ABC news, Clements stated, "The only effective way would be to aerosolize the organisms and this would be much more difficult than for anthrax." He added, "This is mostly due to the fact that, unlike *Bacillus anthracis*, Yersinia do not make spores. Keeping the organism suspended at a high enough concentration, at the right particle size and viable is problematic."[43] But human error and bioterrorism are still concerns. Once infected with plague, a patient is contagious. Any delay or error in diagnosis could increase the odds of additional individuals being exposed to the bacteria. And while a weaponized version of plague may be challenging, that doesn't mean that plague can't be used for bioterror. In fact, plague was part of the possibly first-ever documented case of biological warfare.

During the siege of Caffa in the fourteenth century, the Tartars outside the city walls of Caffa (now called Feodosia, in Ukraine), which had been established by the Genoese and developed into a thriving, cosmopolitan city, began to get ill. They developed swollen lymph nodes under their arms and in their groin and had a foul smell of sickness, oozing fluids, and fever. The pestilence was killing off the Tartars, who then decided to catapult the dead bodies into the city. Because one route of transmission of plague is contact with bodily fluids, those defending Caffa had to handle the many bodies being flung over the wall, which made it highly likely that the plague spread among those inside the walls. When the city's residents began to flee, they made for their boats to return to Italy, bringing the plague with them. Rats carrying fleas infected with the plague also boarded those boats. Whether bubonic or pneumonic, plague is deadly, and treatment must begin as soon as possible. According to the CDC, there are large supplies stockpiled at federal and state level facilities all around the United States that can be sent anywhere in the country within twelve hours.[44] While that's a confident statement, we have seen how slow and

---

43 http://abcnews.go.com/Health/story?id=116771.
44 http://www.bt.cdc.gov/agent/plague/faq.asp.

insufficient emergency assistance from the government has been in the past with other catastrophes. I am less optimistic that our government would be able to transport medications, establish emergency clinics, and distribute those medicines in a timely manner.

Plague Symptoms and Transmission

Septicemic plague is transmitted by contact with infected bodily fluids. Septicemia is when an infection travels through the blood. This is the form of plague that causes hemorrhaging from orifices, and blackened fingers, nose, and toes. It's important not to handle dead animals to avoid both bubonic and septicemic plague. Hunters will need to take extra cautions when handling and processing animals.

When plague is spread from person to person by small water droplets in the air, it's called pneumonic plague. Not only can people get pneumonic plague from other people, but they can also get it from their cat. Cats may pick up plague from eating an infected rodent, such as a mouse, rat, squirrel, or rabbit. If you have a cat, you have a choice: either it's an outside cat, and it doesn't come into the house, or you keep your pet kitty indoors and don't allow it to come in contact with other animals or go outside. Otherwise, cats can become ill and get close to your face, sneeze, or cough, and quickly pass along airborne, pneumonic plague. Something to keep in mind, though, is that rodents often avoid places that smell like cats. Cats are an overall deterrent to rodents and beneficial for keeping diseases like this in check.

Conventional Medical Response

As far as treatment or response for plague, if it's in your area, and you begin feeling symptoms, survival largely depends on how fast you get treatment. Mortality rates, according to CDC, for the United States without treatment is approximately 66 percent, which drops to approximately 11 percent with the use of antibiotics. Even at 11 percent, this is a deadly disease. However, in the PBS series *Rx for Survival*,[45] mortality rates for plague were as follows: bubonic plague,

---

45 http://www.pbs.org/wgbh/rxforsurvival/series/diseases/plague.html.

1 percent to 15 percent with treatment; 50 percent without treatment. Septicemic plague, 40 percent with treatment; 100 percent without treatment. Pneumonic plague, 100 percent without treatment, usually within twenty-four hours.

I could find no definitive mortality rates for pneumonic plague with treatment. But this is a disease that progresses rapidly from a few chills to severe pneumonia with bloody sputum within a day. No time should be lost in getting someone with any form of plague proper treatment, especially pneumonic plague.

Antibiotic Treatment of Plague

There are antibiotics that treat plague, and they're not uncommon in a hospital setting. But for those who are interested in obtaining their own stockpile of antibiotics for their private use, you won't find an equivalent of the preferred antibiotics for plague among aquatic antibiotics. You can, however, obtain the alternatives.

The first choice in antibiotic treatment of plague is streptomycin and gentamicin, neither of which has an aquatic antibiotic counterpart. CDC has posted the information on alternative antibiotics on its website in case neither streptomycin nor gentamicin are available.[46] While CDC suggests administering the medication intravenously, the aquatic equivalents come only in tablet form and should be taken in tablet form. Do not crush the tablet and attempt to administer via an IV. That practice leads to serious, negative outcomes.[47]

For convenience, I have created a table using CDC recommendations for alternative antibiotics for plague, included CDC's recommended dosages for alternative antibiotics for adults, children, and pregnant women, and added their aquatic equivalent. Only those with aquatic equivalents are shown. The CDC recommends selecting only one antibiotic for a duration lasting ten full days, or at least two days after fever subsides.

---

46 http://www.cdc.gov/plague/healthcare/clinicians.html.
47 http://www.sciencedirect.com/science/article/pii/S1078588409000549.

ALTERNATIVE ANTIBIOTIC MEDICATIONS FOR PLAGUE EPIDEMIC/PANDEMIC			
	ALTERNATIVE ANTIBIOTIC	**DOSAGE**	**AQUATIC ANTIBIOTIC EQUIVALENT**
Adults, including pregnant women (See Cautions on page 119)	Doxycycline	100 mg twice daily or 200 mg once daily	Fish Doxy, available in 100 mg tablets or single-use powder
	Ciprofloxacin	400 mg twice daily	Fish Flox, available in 250 mg or 500 mg tablets
Children (See Cautions on page 119)	Doxycycline (for children ≥ 8 years)	Weight < 45 kg: 2.2 mg/kg twice daily (maximum daily dose, 200 mg) Weight ≥ 45 kg: same as adult dose	Fish Doxy, available in 100 mg tablets or single-use powder
	Ciprofloxacin	15 mg/kg twice daily (maximum daily dose, 1 g; can be used with children under 8)	Fish Flox, available in 250 mg or 500 mg tablets

When necessary, either use a powder or crush a tablet to weigh out the correct dosage for a child. There are two steps involved.

1. You need the child's weight in kilograms to get the milligrams per kilograms (mg/kg). Weigh the child either on a scale that measures in kilograms or multiply the child's weight in pounds by 2.2 to convert pounds to kilograms.

2. Then multiple the weight in kilograms by 2.2 again for 2.2 mg/ total weight (kg).

For example, if you have a child who weighed in at 45 kg, multiply this by 2.2, which equals 99 mg. This is essentially the 100 mg dose that adults get. If you have a child who weighs 40 kg, multiply this by 2.2 mg for a total dose of 88 mg. You'll need a digital scale that reads milligrams to get the proper dose. The crushed pill or powder can be mixed in applesauce and fed, as long as the tablet is not a time-release formula. I haven't seen aquatic antibiotics in time-release formulas, so that may be a moot point.

Cautions: There are risks in taking these antibiotics. Pregnant women, children, nursing mothers, and infants would be better off avoiding the need for these medications. But since the illness is so severe and without medication would most likely mean death, it may be better to take the antibiotic medication. Of the two options listed, **the safest choice out of the two antibiotics listed is the ciprofloxacin**. CDC includes doxycycline for women and children, and so I have included it in the chart. I personally would opt for ciprofloxacin only. While they can't be ruled out entirely, there are no known contraindications for ciprofloxacin in pregnant women, and there are known contraindications in doxycycline.

Natural and Herbal Response

As for natural remedies, I know of no good ones. What I can say is that there are a lot of stories about supposed medieval cures for the plague. They range from the absurd, such as leaving a sliced onion in the room of a sick person that will turn black after purifying the room, to the semiplausible, as in the blend known as Four Thieves Vinegar, or in the garlic that grave diggers consumed to ward off illness.

First, the onion. If you cut any onion and leave it out, it'll turn black from the sulphur content. It doesn't absorb the plague or any other illness from the room.

Second, garlic is known to have antibiotic properties and fight infection. It's great stuff, and it couldn't hurt. But I wouldn't trust it alone to shield me from the plague.

Soaking a cloth with Four Thieves Vinegar and using it as a mask over one's mouth and nose might very well cut down on the spread of the disease. Four Thieves Vinegar was supposedly a formula used by four grave robbers who were able to handle corpses and steal from them without becoming sick themselves. This is likely exaggerated, but the herbs that would be steeped in the vinegar were antibacterial, and in combination with a cloth over one's face plus good overall hygiene, especially handwashing, might have provided some protection from infection. It would have done nothing to help someone who was already infected, though.

There are several versions of Four Thieves Vinegar. Jean Valnet, a French aromatherapist, herbalist, and army physician and surgeon, has recorded the following ingredients for Four Thieves Vinegar if you'd like to make your own. If you do make it, I can't promise that you'll be safe to rob graves of plague victims.

Four Thieves Vinegar

- 3 pints white wine vinegar
- Handful of greater wormwood (*Artemisia absinthium*)
- Handful of meadowsweet (*Filipendula ulmaria*)
- Handful of juniper
- Handful of marjoram (*Origanum majorana*)
- Handful of sage
- 50 cloves
- 2 oz. elecampane
- 2 oz. angelica
- 2 oz. rosemary
- 2 oz. horehound (*Marrubium vulgare*)
- 2 oz. camphor (*Cinnamomum camphora*)

Steep these herbs in the vinegar for six weeks, then strain, reserving the liquid. This is now called an acetum, or medicinal vinegar. This could be used in a number of ways, to wet a cloth or face mask to reduce likelihood of infection, or to wash clothing or surfaces. You could also ingest the vinegar, as many of the herbs here are excellent for the respiratory system. Be careful with wormwood if you have any liver issues.

Camphor is not native to the United States and is not something commonly carried in most herb shops. A good substitute would be *Hyssop officinalis*, which is a camphorous plant that's easy to grow here and is a lovely blue flower in the garden. Valnet had a second formula labeled "Marseilles Vinegar or Four Thieves Vinegar."

Marseilles Vinegar

- 40 g greater wormwood
- 40 g lesser wormwood (*Artemisia pontica*)
- 40 g rosemary
- 40 g sage
- 40 g mint

- 40 g rue
- 40 g lavender
- 5 g calamus (*Acorus calamus*)
- 5 g cinnamon
- 5 g clove
- 5 g nutmeg (*Myristica fragrans*)
- 5 g garlic
- 10 g camphor
- 40 g acetic acid
- 2500 g white vinegar

This formula was to be steeped for ten days, except for the camphor and acetic acid, and then strained. Add in the camphor and acetic acid, dissolve the camphor, and strain out again.

There's much good that aromatics can do, though I wouldn't rely on herbs or essential oils solely for plague. I would, however, absolutely use herbal smoke and essential oils in an ionizing diffuser to clean the air. I would also wear an N95 or P100 respirator mask and other appropriate PPE to protect myself.

THE SURPRISE

For this threat, I had no way to use a point system to calculate risk accurately. I could not omit it, however, because new and emerging diseases are part of life on Earth. Having never encountered it before, humanity would have no immunity to this surprise infectious disease. There is no way to know when it will happen or where it will happen. If history is any indicator, one day an unknown illness will emerge.

Cases will trickle in, but few will notice. Eventually, the disease will pick up the pace. It may make the evening news, with reassuring words from the nightly news. Once the number of sick people has reached a critical mass, the caseloads of The Surprise disease will explode with exponential growth. It will spill over borders, rushing through with the violence of a tsunami, washing across borders, and leaving a body count in its wake. News anchors and politicians will repeat talking points overflowing with gravitas, attempt to gain control of the public's perception of the seriousness of the situation, and "look busy."

All that's certain is that a deadly new disease will arise, somewhere, at some time in the future. But there's no indication of when or where it will strike, or how deadly it will be. A surprise, unknown illness has to be a factor, and we have to recognize that it's a certainty a new disease will emerge. Beyond that, however, nothing is certain.

While the nature of this threat defies my simple point system, The Surprise deserves inclusion in this pandemic threat list, if for no other reason than to inspire some thought as to how you would handle such an emergency. How would you respond? While all the other potential pandemic threats have history and modern medicine has treatment protocols, The Surprise won't have any clues to work with. But certainty of a new disease is not justification to put it as a top threat over something like influenza. Be mindful that a totally new disease means that the human population will have no immunity to it, whatever it may be.

The Surprise Overview

Out there, somewhere, is another microorganism. Another virus, another bacteria, another parasite. It may be in the soil, dormant, until awakened by either a change in climate or developers digging into previously undisturbed land. There may be a pathogen in the water of a remote river where humans rarely go, let alone drink, which ends up spreading into millions of water bottles sold when a major corporation comes to exploit this rare and remote river. Perhaps it's a new respiratory virus that leaves us feverish and bleeding from our lungs. Whatever it is, it's out there.

The unknown is a scary proposition. Will antibiotics work? Can a vaccine be made? Are there any herbal medicines that will be effective? What if there's nothing we know of that either treats or prevents the devastation of a previously unknown pathogen to which we have no immunity?

The ugly truth is that sometimes, there isn't anything that can be done. In the early days of a new pandemic, where the cause of the disease is unknown, it's going to take some time for researchers to identify the cause and find a cure. In the meantime, it's likely that physicians and hospitals will be trying everything in their arsenal to prevent the spread of the disease, as well as every type of medication that may possibly kill the infection. Through trial and error, they may stumble on a treatment plan that works most of the time. If the hospitals become overwhelmed, you can bet that people will be looking to any and all alternative practitioners, such as herbalists, aromatherapists, and acupuncturists.

The Surprise Symptoms and Transmission

Risk Factors
Unknown

Symptoms
Unknown

Transmission
Unknown

The Surprise Response

Without specific information about a pathogen, any approach must be broad and widely applicable. Several things to consider are the following:

Improve your current health status. A strong immune system and a healthy body are a head start in avoiding and recovering from almost any infectious disease. There are some exceptions, such as the influenza outbreak in 1918, but being healthy prior to illness will save you more often than not. If you have a chronic illness, do what you can to improve it.

Deter pests: flying, four legged, and two legged. When talking about how disease spreads, certain critters come up repeatedly. Top offenders include insects (mosquitoes, fleas, ticks), rodents (mice, rats, squirrels, rabbits), and other people.

Have a good supply of antibiotic agents, either pharmaceutical or herbal, that can deal with both gram-positive and gram-negative

bacteria. As a new bacterial outbreak progresses, you may hear that it's caused by either gram-positive or gram-negative bacteria. While there may not be a clear course of treatment, at least you would know where to start looking for a potential treatment in your supplies if necessary.

Store herbal antiviral agents. There are precious few available antiviral medications comparable to antibiotics, and it's unlikely you'll be able to obtain them anyway. Herbal antiviral agents are, however, much more available. Again, pay attention to updates for clues, such as if a virus is a DNA or RNA virus, an enveloped virus, or other characteristic information, and look for herbs that have been helpful with other viruses of a similar nature as a starting point for your backup plan.

Be prepared to implement a SIRQ. This is where you go into your home or other secured location, you know the occupants are healthy, and no one goes in or out. How thoroughly this can be implemented is entirely dependent on individual circumstances.

When it comes to infectious disease, population density matters. Obviously, if you have a homestead on twenty acres in a town of less than a thousand people, you have a lot less to worry about from infectious disease than someone in a high-rise apartment in downtown Manhattan.

CHAPTER 6

The Watch List:
Diseases Likely to Spread Postdisaster (Measles, Hantavirus Pulmonary Syndrome, HIV)

Certain diseases have the potential to become pandemics or epidemics after another type of disaster has happened. There are infectious diseases that we have kept at bay only because of our infrastructure. Our current health care system, water treatment systems, and hygiene standards all help keep us healthy and prevent outbreaks of illness. But take that away, and a few diseases stand out as causing major problems, potentially even becoming pandemic diseases.

Measles

Technically, any of the so-called childhood diseases could run wild postdisaster. Here I'm choosing to focus on measles, since it seems to be the one that gets the most attention when there's an outbreak.

Measles has been "eradicated" in the United States, except for when someone travels to the United States who has contracted measles elsewhere. We recently had an outbreak at Disneyland in California. There were 147 people who became ill, and no one died. CDC believes that the most likely scenario is that a traveler from overseas brought measles into the United States.[48]

Most of those who became ill were not vaccinated previously. Sometimes, vaccination does not offer complete protection. There's about 10 percent of the population that even after receiving two measles vaccinations do not produce the anticipated antibodies. Also, over time, people can lose immunity to measles from vaccinations. After this outbreak, arguments over vaccinations, between those who choose not to have their children vaccinated and those who support mandatory vaccinations, broke out all over social media and the Internet. From social networking sites like Twitter and Facebook to blogs and news media comment sections, the remarks bore little resemblance to conversation and dialogue. There were nasty, vile, accusatory statements from both sides. In the end, nothing was resolved, but it did demonstrate a massive shift in public perception about measles.

Today, the thought of a measles outbreak is frightening. Ask random people, "What is measles?" and you're likely to be told that it's a horrible disease that kills children. To a certain extent, that's true. But this is a far cry from the public's perception of measles in the 1960s, when measles was nothing more alarming than chicken pox. It was seen as a very uncomfortable childhood illness that almost everyone went through. Granted, it was absolute misery for a few days, but it was something you just put up with and got through. It didn't carry the panic that it does today. Considering that we have "eradicated" measles in the United States, and we have a vaccine for it, it seems odd to me that we would have more panic now than when it was prevalent.

If we take a look at measles prior to 1962 (the measles vaccine became available in 1963), we find that the United States had three million to four million people who became infected with measles each year. Of those, approximately four hundred to five hundred died. Some would be children, and some of those deaths would be adults. Unfortunately, CDC doesn't publish the breakdown of children versus adult deaths for measles. If we take the lower figure of three million infected, and the highest number of five hundred deaths, this gives us the highest

---

48 http://www.cdc.gov/measles/cases-outbreaks.html.

percentage possible for a mortality rate of 0.017 percent. I would suggest that *under first-world conditions*, the risk of fatal outcome is far overblown and causes an unnecessary amount of panic and division.

To be fair, in underdeveloped countries where there's great poverty and hunger, measles remains a leading cause of death for children. It's not that measles is more virulent overseas but that those infected are suffering from severe, nutritional deficiencies before contracting the measles virus, especially vitamin A. Standard procedure for measles in these regions includes vitamin A drops, but even WHO admits that this isn't nearly as effective as not being deficient in vitamin A in the first place. But what if we were to suddenly be facing great poverty and hunger? Isn't that why we prep?

If we were to face a calamity with disruptions in both food and medical supplies reaching local stores and medical offices, we would eventually see childhood diseases become more prevalent. While it may not be highly lethal in times of plenty, it's at all times highly infectious. If it makes it to your region and you have either never had measles or been vaccinated, you're at risk. If tough times have led to food shortages and malnutrition, we must anticipate that we'll see more deaths from measles.

Recognizing measles isn't difficult. It may start out like a flu with cough, sore throat, and achiness, and there will also be white spots in the mouth, fever, conjunctivitis, and of course, the famous red, flat, blotchy rash. Measles incubates in the body for ten to fourteen days, and the patient is infectious about four days before the onset of the rash until about four days after the onset of the rash, or eight days.

The key here is to maintain good health through good nutrition. While it's easy to just buy buckets of dehydrated "survival food," and such products have their place, you must consider nutritional value and the overall health to be gained from your food storage. During emergencies, you need every advantage you can get. High-sodium camping foods might be fine for the bug-out bag, but not for everyday food storage that you intend on keeping. Making your own long-term food storage is the way to go, either through pressure canning or dehydrating, and especially from your own garden. It's less expensive overall, and you can control the ingredients.

To take it a step further, know your wild edibles. Go foraging with a solid field guide for your region, like one of the Peterson's field guides, or *The Forager's Harvest*, by Samuel Thayer. Wild plants tend to be more vigorous than cultivated ones and pack more nutrition. This will become especially important if you have to abandon your food storage for any reason.

Hantavirus

While one form of hanta viral infection was mentioned briefly in the VHF section, that's not what we typically see in the United States. We're far more likely to see hantavirus pulmonary syndrome.

Hantavirus is spread by rodents. While the virus doesn't make these host animals sick, they can spread it anywhere they make their homes. Deer mice, white-footed mice, cotton rats, and rice rats can carry hantavirus. According to CDC, transmission can happen whenever fresh urine, droppings, saliva, or nesting materials (which may have these on them) are stirred up. The droplets become aerosoled into the air and pass into humans through airborne transmission. Transmission can also occur through a bite, touching a contaminated surface and then touching one's mouth, or eating food contaminated by infected rodents. The hantavirus strains in the United States are not transmitted person to person, through kissing or other close contact.

Hantavirus pulmonary syndrome may be especially problematic to preppers and survivalists, which is why it's included here. It already exists in both the United States and Canada. Though it's more prevalent in the western states, hantavirus does exist in the eastern states as well. But it isn't something we have to wait to come to the United States from elsewhere. It's already here, and the kinds of activities most likely to spread hanta are things preppers, survivalists, and homesteaders do with some frequency; for example, opening and cleaning out unused buildings, like cabins or campers used as bugging-out locations. Other activities include camping, hiking, and cleaning in areas where mice may have found their way into a home.

This is a serious virus that has a mortality rate of 38 percent,[49] and there's no specific treatment. It comes in two stages. The early stage has some fairly nondescript symptoms that could seem like a dozen other illnesses, such as fever, muscle aches, dizziness, chills, nausea, diarrhea, and vomiting. The only clue that it might be hanta at this stage would be that the muscle aches are in the large muscle groups, such as thighs, hips, back, and shoulders. The late stage begins four to ten days after the early stage and brings severe tightness and difficulty breathing as the lungs fill with fluids, sometime causing the patient to, in effect, drown.

The standard treatment in a hospital setting would include intubation and oxygen to assist breathing during the worst stages of the illness. This seems to work better the sooner this level of care can be started. When the patient is already in such distress, intubation and oxygen become less effective.

From an herbal perspective, I don't know anything that's effective against this virus specifically. But there may be herbs to help with the symptoms. Expectorants and any herbs that are beneficial for the symptoms of pneumonia may provide some comfort. Pleurisy root (*Asclepias tuberosa*), thyme, hyssop, clove, mullein, marshmallow root, licorice, garlic, elecampane, coltsfoot, lemon, honey, and cayenne are all options for comfort care.

Think about kinds of circumstances where it's imperative to bug out, because I can easily envision hantavirus spreading with people squatting in unused spaces, without a way to clean them safely. If you have a bug-out location, go there with some frequency. Be a presence. Clean any sign of rodent activity immediately. If you have a camper or cabin that's been dormant for a while and has signs of rodent activity, consider getting a professional team to come in and clean it. If you must do it yourself, do not attempt cleaning it without wearing PPE, perhaps a Tyvek suit, gloves, and most importantly, a face mask to prevent inhalation of the virus. Remove any obvious signs of rodents, such as droppings or bedding, and secure it away from your family. Use a pump sprayer to apply a bleach and water solution on all surfaces, and

---

49 http://www.cdc.gov/hantavirus/hps/symptoms.html.

allow to dry. I would use a 1:10 ratio of 1 part bleach to 10 parts water. Make sure to clean all surfaces thoroughly. Rodents bring all manner of disease. Do whatever you can to prevent their presence in your home. Be on the watch for them in sheds and barns as well.

One of the best deterrents for mice is peppermint. They hate it. Plant it everywhere. Of course, many gardeners hate it too, since it can take over wherever it's planted. But if you're going to be absent for any length of time from your secondary or even tertiary locations, then perhaps an overgrowth of peppermint to deter rodents and other pests might just be the perfect solution.

Human Immunodeficiency Virus (HIV)

No discussion of pandemics would be complete without human immunodeficiency virus. Of all the diseases mentioned here, there's no other pathogen, bacterial or viral, poised to do as much damage to the human population postdisaster than HIV.

HIV is a current pandemic, though many of us have allowed it to fall into the background of our lives. It isn't nearly so scary today as it was in the 1980s. There isn't nearly as much attention to it today either. In fact, more people lose their minds in panic over diseases like measles than HIV. This is, in my humble opinion, totally insane.

The fact remains that even though it's 2016, we still have no cure for acquired immunodeficiency syndrome, which is the ultimate fate of those infected with HIV. It's a 100 percent death sentence. If a person has HIV, it isn't long before that person can spread it to others. In fact, there's about a two-week to four-week or two-week to six-month (depending on your source) incubation period before HIV antibodies can even be detected in a laboratory test, and long before any symptoms may arise. Some people will have an initial reaction to the infection within two to four weeks similar to the flu. The infected person then enters a latent period where he or she is asymptomatic. Unfortunately, the person is still capable of spreading the disease.

Without treatment, life expectancy is around three years. But in that time, a single infected person who may not have any idea that he or she is infected could spread it to countless others through sharing needles and unprotected sexual intercourse. Technically, any contact of bodily fluids to an opening to the body, through birth, through sex, through an open wound, and so forth, can spread it. But intercourse and sharing needles are the two most likely ways to spread HIV.

So why, if there's a 100 percent mortality rate without treatment, do we get all in a tizzy over measles, but not worry about HIV? Unfortunately, we've learned to accept HIV into our society. We rely on testing to identify those infected to get them proper care, but also to stop, we hope, the spread of this disease. We rely on medications to help those who are infected, such as the famed basketball star Magic Johnson, who has lived with HIV for over twenty years without developing AIDS, to keep them healthy and living their lives as close to normal as possible. In Johnson's case and in many others like him, the key has been a combination of medications that has kept his viral load from increasing. This prevents the development of the disease in that patient, though the person is still contagious.

But in a postdisaster situation, those medications would no longer be available. Not only would the medications be gone, but access to medical testing for HIV would be too. Within a few years, we would begin to see deaths from AIDS. Consider that right now, one in every eight people currently infected with HIV doesn't even know he or she has it. Half of all children, meaning teenagers, who have HIV don't even know they have it. They may live for a few years with absolutely no symptoms, engaging in all manner of normal human behavior, and pass along the disease to others, who will also not know they were infected.

We have become complacent about HIV over the past decade. As our understanding of treating it grew and life expectancy increased, HIV became less scary. If we were to face a real "end of the world as we know it" situation, such as an EMP or other major catastrophe where rebuilding would take years, deadly, stealthy, untreated HIV and AIDS may still be the largest threat to human health we ever face.

CHAPTER 7

Pandemic Preparation 201:
Actionable Steps

So far, we've covered a lot of background information, including lessons to be learned from a current pandemic; disease threats that could become the next great pandemic, including their symptoms, conventional and alternative care, and transmission; and a "crash course" of general pandemic and postdisaster health information.

While this is already plenty of good information, it doesn't exactly say what to do. That's what this chapter is all about. My goal here is to provide clear, actionable steps that you can start on today.

Naturally, your specific plans for pandemic preparation are going to depend on your unique circumstances. There are different concerns for people in urban, suburban, and rural areas. You may be bugging out. You may be bugging in or sheltering in place, where your circumstances dictate that you'll stay in your primary location for the duration of the crisis. You may be an expert prepper with years of food and water storage, and twenty different ways to defend your home. You might, however, be brand new to preparedness and feel a bit overwhelmed by everything.

For those feeling overwhelmed, let me start by saying that when you prepare for one event, you actually are prepping for multiple events. No matter the crisis, the things humans require for survival don't change. We require water, food, and shelter. This means clean water that won't make us sick, nutrient- and calorie-dense foods to keep us healthy, and some protection from the elements. This shelter could be anything from a tarp and a wool sweater and socks to a lean-to, commercially made tent, cabin, or modern home. To improve our situation, we might want to add to that list energy (electricity, gas, wood, etc.) and security (gates, cameras, defensive capabilities). We also need to cover other aspects of surviving a long-term emergency, such as financial preparedness and medical preparedness.

Let's get started.

Logistics of Bugging In or Out during a Pandemic

Here's the million-dollar question: should you shelter in place, or should you get out of dodge? There are many pros and cons to each, and there really is no good, single, definitive answer for all people. I will, however, provide a list of things to consider when making your own plans, as well as my own personal criteria for determining when it's time to get out.

First, here's a list of variables to consider when analyzing your own situation:

- Do you live in a highly populated area? Population density matters!
- Do you have a suitable location in which to retreat?
- If you were to leave, could you get there on foot if you had to?
- Could you get there on foot in all seasons?
- If your answer is no to either of the two previous points, do you have a plan for getting there other than driving on major highways?
- Do you have supplies there to last you at least a year?
- How dependent are you on utilities (water, electricity, gas, etc.)?
- Do you have a way to defend your home?
- Do you have a way to pay your bills if you suddenly relocated?
- Do you have time saved up at work if you needed to take some extended time off?

This doesn't even get into whether you may have family members in the area or whether they would be willing to leave with you. But this should be enough to begin a rational dialogue about whether you really have what you would need to bug out effectively during a pandemic.

If you must stay where you are or are already in a more sparsely populated town, one of the most important things you can do is to build your survival community. You won't be able to survive all on your own. You stand a far better chance of ensuring food and water security if multiple people in your neighborhood all start storing their food, water, and other necessary supplies. You'll be able to group together for mutual defense against looters and anyone who wishes to bring harm or control your area. But only if you organize and plan for it.

Personally, I look back on the wealthier families of medieval Europe and how they avoided the entire ugly business of the plague by leaving the city. They did what the peasants had no chance of doing and, as a consequence, the latter suffered miserably. But in our modern world where so many people are comfortable in their lives and preparedness isn't even on their radar, retreating to an area with a lower population density makes absolute sense to me.

This will also require planning. You must decide on where you believe you're safest. Is this a place you would want to relocate to permanently, effectively negating the need to "bug out" later or even allowing you the opportunity to secure an even more remote secondary location? What supplies do you feel comfortable leaving there? Who in the area can keep an eye on the place for you in your absence?

Financial preparedness will play a big role in your choices. If you had to leave, how will you meet your financial obligations? Let's assume that totally drug-resistant tuberculosis came to the United States, and it was running rampant throughout schools, hospitals, office buildings, shopping malls, and any other place where people congregate. If you wanted to distance your family from this, could you afford to up and leave?

If it's important to you to have this option, you need to start thinking about either finding work near your bug-out location, especially if you plan to move there permanently, or finding a way to earn money without being tied to a particular area. This may mean owning rental properties and having a property management company take care of them while you live wherever you choose. It may mean that you and your boss work out an arrangement to telecommute. It might mean starting your own Internet-based business.

At the very least, save up your sick days and personal days. While everyone needs a break, and you should enjoy your vacation time, don't waste sick days and personal days to stay home just because you want a day off. Unless you have a situation where you lose your time off if you don't use it, save up your sick time. Let it accrue. If there's a pandemic, and you call in sick to bug out, no one is going to question it.

Whatever it takes, if you want to have the ability to relocate, then you must address how you'll support yourself financially. You could just pack up and go, and that would be understandable. But you can bet that if you owe any money on a car, mortgage, school loan, credit card, and so forth, the lending institution isn't going to give you a "pandemic waiver" and let you skip out on payments. Eventually, the crisis will come to an end, and there will be a price to pay, plus interest. To that end, you'll have far more freedom to live where you wish and relocate if you don't carry debt. The less debt you have, the more freedom of movement you have.

For those who are going to leave, and know that they're going to leave, the only real question is *how do you know when it's time?*

I used to think that if I heard a verified news report that a particularly deadly, infectious disease was found within fifty miles of my home, that would be my family's trigger to leave. But after watching the media go silent on both Ebola and enterovirus D68 (EV D68) at about the same time—even though I knew from sources in my local medical community that there were still ongoing infections of EV D68—I'm no longer willing to rely solely on that metric to determine when it's time to leave.

The first thing you need to make a good decision about this is good information. The only problem is that you can't depend on the government to provide good information. This isn't about being afraid of the government but recognizing that the government's interests during a pandemic (or any emergency) are not the same as your interests.

Enterovirus D68

Enterovirus D68 is one of many enteroviruses. EV D68 has the same symptoms and is transmitted the same way as other respiratory viruses, and is a common cause of summer and early autumn colds. However, EV D68 flared up in 2014 in a nationwide outbreak, specifically targeting children. Some children developed asthma-like symptoms, resulting in serious illness and in some cases, death. Many were infected, with hospitals in the Midwest running out of beds and rerouting patients to other hospitals. This virus left some children with partial, possibly permanent, paralysis of the limbs. These cases had a mutated strain of EV D68, similar to a distant relation to another, more well-known enterovirus, polio.

The government's primary goal prior to a disaster like a deadly pandemic disease is to maintain the status quo. The government doesn't want people rushing to stores to stock up, to store water, to get cash out of the bank, or to stand in line at the gas station to fill up spare cans to run the generator. The government at all levels, federal, state, and local, wants to prevent panic and maintain order. That may include blocking access to roads, enforcing curfews, and quarantines. Bottom line, if you wait too long, your decision whether to leave or not will be made for you.

The government is never going to say, "Hey, if you were thinking of leaving, this is your best chance. Because tomorrow, we're going to shut down part of the interstate to help curb the spread of this disease." Instead, you'll have to be alert and have other sources of information.

After talking with a few trusted friends who have served in war zones about practical and tactical issues that had been weighing on my mind, and really listening to what they had to say, I have had to rethink my current living arrangements, my distance to my bug-out location, and the reality of attempting to bug out for a crisis. Something I hadn't considered, and I'm grateful for having it pointed out to me, is that if you wait too long to bug out, and you're the only one on the road, you're a target. A big, fat target on four wheels trucking down the highway, just asking to get picked off.

It doesn't matter that you've got your ultimate bug-out vehicle with spare gas and a trailer behind to tow your bigger gear, and a luggage rack above to carry even more supplies, a custom push bar, and your map with a primary, secondary, and tertiary route all highlighted and waterproofed. It doesn't matter. Understand that you'll stand out. If you've waited too long, and you're the only thing moving on the road, you're going to be a giant target. You'll be better off sheltering in place. Or, if you absolutely must go, then go on foot, and stay off the main roads.

I thought about this and the reality of trying to hoof it all the way to our bug-out location, in the winter, with two kids. It's not practical. It's certainly a poor tactical choice. So we've made the decision to take all necessary measures to simply relocate to our bug-out location full-time. Our plans then would be to shelter in place instead. Until that time, the following are the criteria we've established for determining when our family would leave, which makes sense for our circumstances:

Is it winter? Forget it, shelter in place. Is it any time other than winter? See below.

Pay attention to the news. If the news reports a case of a deadly, infectious disease in your region, assume that it's not the only case. Get bags and vehicles packed, and watch for at least two other signs or news of other cases. This plus two other signs, and my family is going on "vacation."

Pay attention to banks and ATMs. If there are a lot of ATMs running out of cash, or there are longer lines than usual at the bank, especially if the branch has to call around to see if other branches can cash larger checks, it may mean that the cash flow is being limited by the local Federal Reserve, which sends cash by armored vehicle on a schedule to all other banks and their branches in the area. If this becomes a trend for more than a couple of days, this is cause for concern.

Pay attention to store shelves. Even if you buy in bulk once a month, or you get your meat from a local farmer once a year, if you're suspicious that a pandemic is on the way, get out and do some reconnaissance. Are stores having trouble keeping shelves stocked? If so, find out why. Is this because others are sensing the tension or because there may be an issue with resupply? For example, for a resupply issue, consider food manufacturing and shipping slowing down because of people calling in sick.

General tension. If it's general tension, make any final preparations to leave on a moment's notice, but sit tight. It may just be tension because of something else entirely, like an election or a divisive news story.

Resupply issues. If it's because of a resupply issue, get out of dodge ASAP, preferably quietly, at night. There's no need to announce that you've vacated your home.

Pay attention to gas pumps. This is for the same reason you're watching the store shelves.

Pay attention to other sources of information. Sources such as HealthMap.org, which maps reported outbreaks of disease, can give a better idea of what's going on around the world and around the country.

Pay attention to social media. One thing that Facebook, Twitter, and G+ have been able to do successfully is connect people around the country and all over the world. Find a few trusted individuals and check in with each other regularly. Not all day long, but designate a time. Find out if the news reports in their neck of the woods sound like yours.

Drive by the local hospitals. Does anything look out of the ordinary? Drive past the emergency room entrance, not just the main entrance. Can you see if the waiting room is packed? If so, is this a time of year you could reasonably expect to see a packed waiting room? If this is out of the ordinary, it's probably time to leave.

Pay attention to the stock market. When the news was still reporting on the Ebola pandemic, the stock market felt the pinch, and this happened without an outbreak even happening here.

Pay attention to the American Society of Hospital Pharmacists' current medication shortage list. It's on their website, www.ASHP. org. Be on the lookout for antibiotics, antivirals, and common things to keep people hydrated, such as saline. They publish a list once a week.

Are your friends prepping? Finally, if friends who typically have no interest in prepping suddenly start asking you serious questions about prepping, it may be time to leave.

There's never going to be an easy, foolproof way to tell that "it's time" to bug out. The trick is to get out early and get out quietly, before others catch on and the road ahead for you and your family turns into a parking lot of other people's cars, with everyone trying to leave at the same time.

Self-Imposed Reverse Quarantine

The most basic element of pandemic preparedness is understanding how to effectively execute a SIRQ. So what is a SIRQ, and how does it differ from a regular quarantine?

Normally, a quarantine is an imposed separation by an authority on someone or a group of people when the authority suspects that a person or persons are infectious with a disease that threatens the larger community. The person or group are separated and observed for signs of illness. A SIRQ, in contrast, is where a person or a group of people voluntarily separate themselves to protect their own health from an infectious disease in the community.

The basic steps of implementing a SIRQ include choosing your location, determining and securing the perimeter, and stocking your location with supplies to outlast the pandemic.

Choosing Your Location

For most people, the SIRQ plan will revolve around either their home or a secondary location, often called a bug-out location (BOL). If you live in a rural location, such as on your own homestead, it makes sense to base your SIRQ in your home. If you live in a city or suburb, having a BOL and recognizing when to retreat to it is a smart plan. Unfortunately, when it comes to infectious disease, population density matters.

If you do have a BOL, be sure to be a presence there on a somewhat regular, frequent basis. Abandoned cabins are susceptible to infestations of mice and spiders, and who knows what else. They can also attract two-legged pests. Your BOL should be an ongoing concern, and look like one. Otherwise, you might have an unpleasant surprise waiting for you upon arrival.

Make it a point to get to know the neighbors in the area and stay on good terms. Knowing that there are good people keeping an eye on your place when you're not there is another layer of insurance. For example, one weekend when my husband drove up to our BOL to work on it, the neighbor called him on his cell phone to ask if there was supposed to be anyone there. Of course, it was my husband's SUV the neighbor saw pull in, and they met up the next day for a beer. That kind of courtesy can be worth more than gold in an emergency.

If you can't purchase a more remote property at the present time, perhaps you can work out an arrangement in advance with a family member or close friend who is situated in a better location than you currently are. If not, I'll cover some strategies for a SIRQ in more populated areas, including ideas for when public services and utilities are interrupted. Examples include waste removal, municipal water supplies, and intermittent electrical service.

Determining and Securing the Perimeter

What Is a Perimeter?
The perimeter is your protection. It's the barrier behind which you and your healthy group remain, and beyond which the potential of infection exists. The ability to secure that perimeter is crucial. If an infectious disease that disrupts services and causes food shortages is going to be in your area for more than a few weeks, you can expect hungry, desperate people to ignore any imposed quarantine the government may impose and go searching for food and any other supplies that might make this crisis less miserable.

Urban Concerns
Depending on your circumstances, your perimeter may be predetermined for you. If you live in a city apartment, the walls of your unit are your perimeter, with entry points, or weak points, at the door and windows. You may wish to get some plywood to board up your windows if you're on lower floors where someone could potentially breach your perimeter through the glass. You can do several things to shore up a door, from securing it with solid locks, "C" brackets, and two-by-four boards or steel bars across the bottom and top third of the door, or even a heavy piece of furniture if need be.

The boards or bars in brackets across the door will do a few things. First, if you have to get out that door, it's a lot faster and easier to slide them out of the brackets than to move heavy furniture. While this door can still be breached, it'll take time to break it down, cause a lot of noise, and draw lots of attention. Those are usually things criminals try to avoid. It'll also give you plenty of time to either escape out another exit or prepare to confront the intruder.

The Importance of Blackout Curtains

If you live higher up in a building, entry through the window may not be your primary concern. But after securing the door, you should still be concerned about your windows. This is especially true if the electrical supply in your area becomes intermittent because of people not showing up to work due to illness. You may have some backup power, rechargeable lighting, or perhaps candles. In a city experiencing a power outage, however, any light coming from your unit will stand out like a sore thumb.

Blackout curtains solve this and several other problems. Blackout curtains prevent the light inside from being seen outside, but also prevent the light outside from being seen inside. If you've put various family or group members on a rotational shift so that someone is awake and alert around the clock, those individuals will need all the help they can to get a good rest during daylight hours. No matter how much of a night owl a person may be, and I count myself as one, most people do not sleep well during the day. Proper sleep becomes even more important when you must keep your immune response strong. Also, if you can't designate a room away from the rest of the family for the night-shift folks to sleep, consider some foam ear plugs, and try to keep noise to a minimum. If there are small children involved, this is going to be impossible. Just do the best that you can.

An Extra Pair of Eyes: Surveillance Cameras

No matter what your situation is, a downtown apartment or a log cabin in the mountains, having a camera that lets you view who's on the other side of the door before you get close to it is a great idea. If you're expecting someone to join your group, you can view, from a safe distance, the person ringing the bell or knocking. If it's your group member, great. Let the individual in and lead him or her to the quarantine room where he or she will stay until it's no longer likely that the individual is sick. If not, you have a chance to preview the unknown persons and ascertain whether they're armed and looking to cause trouble.

Suburban Concerns

If you live in your own home in a small city or a suburb, this opens the options up to include a small yard. As the saying goes, good fences make good neighbors. In this case, we're not talking about a short picket fence. We are talking about a privacy fence. Depending on how your property is laid out, this privacy fence may funnel anyone who wishes to enter your home to a single, preselected door. The yard surrounding the building may be your perimeter. If weather permits and you can secure your yard, it may make good decontamination, quarantine, and isolation areas.

A decontamination area is when a person who has been beyond the perimeter, but has been wearing personal protective equipment, can safely remove the PPE, wash, change into clean clothing, and so on, prior to rejoining the group inside the perimeter.

Quarantine versus Isolation

A quarantine area is where an individual is isolated and observed for any signs of illness. If the incubation period for the disease has passed and there are no signs of illness, it's likely safe to permit the person to join the group inside the perimeter. Normally, it's a government agency enforcing the quarantine. However, as the property owner and the authority in this circumstance, you decide who gains entry to your home.

Isolation is when someone has developed signs and symptoms of the disease. The person is kept away from the healthy people in the group. A large, quality tent can be used for quarantine or isolation area. When this is done indoors, it's often called a "sickroom."

This assumes that being outdoors will not cause further injury or hasten the illness. If your only yard is on the front lawn and visible to the entire neighborhood, the neighbors might grab their torches and pitchforks and storm your castle for keeping sick people close to their homes. This is best for those who have some privacy. Otherwise, quarantine and isolation may have to happen in a designated space within the perimeter, such as a basement or some rarely used but ventilated space.

Rural Concerns

If you live in a rural area, your perimeter can be substantially larger depending on how many acres your property is and if you have outbuildings, livestock, a garden, and so forth. Your perimeter may be rather small, just the main house and a section in the backyard, or it may include some outbuildings like barns and sheds. You may need to have a plan for protecting livestock, either bringing them into your perimeter or extending your perimeter out to include those outbuildings.

No matter where you live, the larger your perimeter, the more challenging it'll be to keep it secure. This can be helped with extra fencing, cameras, extra people, elevated observation posts, guard dogs, and alarm systems. Alarm systems can be as high tech or as low tech as you wish them to be. For some, loud homemade alarms set off by tripwire or a barking dog may be the only alarm system in place. These low-tech systems can be tripped by local wildlife, but are also affordable on any budget. For others, gadgets, cameras, silent alarms, and computerized systems may be the answer. These are sophisticated and allow the homeowner to view from a protected command center what has tripped the alarm. These systems are, however, vulnerable to power failures, cut wires, and other technical problems. Each approach has pros and cons, and every situation is unique.

In addition to barricades and perimeter alarms, if a pandemic has progressed long enough that civil unrest has erupted, it's usually wise to learn how to use some form of defensive weapon. Firearms are ideal for this, as you can most easily maintain your distance from any intruder with them. Be mindful of the risks involved when firing in the home. I suggest taking an additional firearms training course specifically for home defense. If for some reason an intruder is capable of breaching your perimeter or door, and you don't have your chosen firearm with you, it's also a good idea to have studied some form of martial arts, such as Krav Maga. You may risk infection from being so close, but it's more important to deal with the immediate threat, an attacker, in this scenario.

Neatness Matters

Some intruders are less obvious. For example, rodents, ticks, fleas, and mosquitoes bring disease easily, quickly, and silently. The best thing to do is to deter them. Cleaning up, preventing standing water, keeping grass trimmed low, and planting herbs and flowers that these pests dislike will help keep your SIRQ successful.

Herbal Allies and Plant Helpers

There's one herb that I know of that will grow almost anywhere and repels just about every pest you can think of. It's peppermint. I know, it's not exotic. It's just plain old peppermint. But it's amazing stuff. Mice hate it. Ants hate it. Ticks hate it. Even mosquitoes find it repulsive. Yet, to us, it smells clean and is reminiscent of candy, bubblegum, or toothpaste. Of course, it grows just about anywhere, which means it'll probably spread to places you don't want it to spread. What it brings is sharp little branches and leaves rich in essential oil that mice and other pests hate.

Other helpful plants are cedar trees (red and yellow), lemon balm (*Melissa officinalis*), basil (*Ocimum basilicum*), and marigolds. By marigolds, I need to be specific that both the genus *Tagetes* (French, Mexican, and African marigolds) and *Calendula officinalis* (pot marigold) are helpful in repelling unwanted flies and mosquitoes. I've grown them both, and it seems that they both work reasonably well at keeping pests out of the general area where they're planted while still attracting pollinators. I plant calendula and basil with my tomato and bean plants in the garden. If you're using these plants to repel potentially disease-carrying insects, you can always put them in pots along your steps, decks, flower boxes, and so on.

When it comes to bug repellents, DEET has been the gold standard for effectiveness. Unfortunately, it also comes with well-documented risks, and it should not be used on or around children. On the plus side, several essential oils make excellent bug repellents. The only drawback may be that you need to reapply more often. Still, that's a small price to pay to avoid the potential burns and seizures that may happen as a result of DEET. Another good note to mention is that the CDC has declared that lemon eucalyptus oil (*Corymbia citriodora*) is as effective as DEET. Not all oils are safe for children, and some kids have a hard time with any eucalyptus oil. In that case, substitute rosalina (*Melaleuca ericifolia*), which is similar in action to the lemon eucalyptus oil.

I make a blend of the following essential oils to repel potentially disease-carrying insects:

- Cedarwood (*Cedrus deodara*), 35 drops
- Lemon eucalyptus or rosalina, 15 drops
- Rose geranium bourbon (*Pelargonium x asperum*), 15 drops
- Peppermint, 15 drops
- Basil, 10 drops
- Rosemary (leave out if for children), 5 drops
- Tea tree (*Melaleuca alternifolia*), 5 drops

Blend this into 1 ounce of olive oil, and rub onto the skin. You could also add these oils to one-half ounce of witch hazel, one-fourth ounce of grape seed oil, and one-fourth ounce aloe vera gel. This makes a spray that can be applied to both skin and clothing without leaving large oil stains. The spray will have to be reapplied more frequently than the olive oil, as it will lack the staying power of the heavier oil.

Stock Your Location with Supplies to Outlast the Pandemic

There are so many variables here, that makes it impossible to provide a master list that would work in every situation. I focus on the commonalities and branch out from there.

No matter who or where you're implementing your SIRQ, you'll require food, water, shelter, energy, and security. Shelter and security were addressed above when choosing your locations, and determining and securing your perimeter. Now, we need to address food, water, and energy to last until order can be restored. Something often left off this list, but becomes obvious for pandemic preparation, is medical supplies.

There are two big questions: how long will the pandemic last, and what supplies do you specifically need to stock.

Unfortunately, there's no way to know for certain just how long a pandemic might last. For example, the Spanish flu came in two waves with a break in the middle. It lasted from January 1918 through December 1920, nearly three years. The current Ebola pandemic is well into its second year. Other infections may become endemic, and we may just have to learn to cope with a new normal, such as in the prospect of totally drug-resistant MRSA.

Food Storage

Many prepping guidelines recommend a year's worth of food storage. I suggest that, for a pandemic, a year's worth of food storage is not enough. I would aim for three to five years. Some preppers may feel that's unreasonable and over the top. But when you look at how long a pandemic can last, these are events that typically span multiple years.

I can hear the objections. "That's too much, I wouldn't have any place to store all that." Or, "I live on a farm and grow most of what I need. All I need is a year's worth of supplies." That's fine. Space is absolutely a consideration, and the ability to grow your own is invaluable. But if you were to become ill during this pandemic, and you weren't able to get to your fields and work or care for your animals, then you may appreciate having that extra food on hand. I do recognize that for those new to prepping, the idea of storing up to five years' worth of food is overwhelming. This is what I consider ideal based on the long-term nature of a pandemic. It's not like an isolated storm. It's not an earthquake. Almost always, pandemics are long-term events. Don't let the large scale of what I personally think is the right amount of food storage stop you from taking action.

Start with planning for two weeks' worth of shelf-stable foods. Then expand that to a month. From there, it shouldn't be too difficult to expand that one month into three months' worth of food storage. Increase your food storage to six months. That's a significant achievement, as it prepares you for a multitude of other scenarios, not just pandemics.

I encourage you to have a variety of foods in your food-storage plans. Freeze-dried foods are expensive, but have a great shelf life and take up little space. The same can be said for properly stored, home-dehydrated foods. Though the shelf life is shorter than freeze-dried, the expense of dehydrating and storing food from your garden is significantly lower than buying freeze-dried. Home canning, when done properly, provides another great option for long-term food storage. You can pressure can meats, vegetables, and whole meals, like chili. The great thing about home canning and home dehydrating is that you can control everything that goes into your food, allowing you to create long-term, shelf-stable food that's healthy, free of artificial ingredients, nutrient rich, and far more affordable than buckets of freeze-dried foods. But don't ignore those ready-made food storage buckets entirely. They're a great way to create a lot of food storage instantly.

Water Storage

If you have a private well, you may not need to worry about this so much. But if your well is run on an electrical pump and there's suddenly no power because of low employee turnout for electrical providers, you should consider a backup, either a solar-powered pump or a hand pump.

For the rest of us who depend on municipal water supplies, water storage becomes more of a necessity. The standard guideline for storing water is 1 gallon of water per person per day.

When you store water, however, you run the risk of growing bacteria. To prevent bacteria growth:

- Store water in an opaque container to block out all light.
- Store water in a cool area where the temperature is stable.
- If you store water out of the faucet, it will already have chlorine in it, which will prevent bacteria from growing.
- If you store rainwater, you will have to purify it somehow to make sure that you don't ingest something harmful.

Options for purification include water filters, chlorine bleach, iodine, and boiling. There are many more. I opted for a Berkey filter. I bought the largest one available, and I love it. While I primarily use it for our drinking and cooking water, since our municipal water tastes strongly of metals and chlorine, it would work wonderfully if we had to filter rainwater instead. You can also make your own DIY Berkey filters with two 5-gallon buckets, a circular cutter, and simple hardware that you can find at your local hardware store. All you'll have to buy are the filters, which can be cleaned and reused multiple times before needing to be replaced.

If you have to leave in a hurry, my choice would be to keep something like the Sawyer Mini Water Filtration System in your bug-out bag because it can filter one hundred thousand gallons of water before needing to be replaced. The only other filter that comes close in ease of use is the Lifestraw Personal Water Filter, which can filter one thousand gallons of water before needing to be replaced.

For those who want to store water indoors, especially those who have little space available, the choice of container is critical. We have used 7-gallon tanks with spigots, one for each member of the household, representing a week's worth of water. But we couldn't stack them, and there's only so much floor space we can take up with water tanks. WaterBOBs, an emergency, collapsible water container that you fill in the bathtub, weren't going to be adequate by themselves either. The best option I've come across is the WaterBrick. These interlocking containers stack and lock together like Legos. They hold 3.5 gallons each, making them much lighter to move around than the 7-gallon ones I had been using. And of course, these can be stacked several rows high without risk of them falling over or leaking.

A gallon of water per day is not nearly as much as one might think. This has to be used for drinking, cooking, bathing, washing dishes, and washing clothing. This becomes especially important when it comes to hygiene and cleanliness in the home during a pandemic. So, while survival is possible on a gallon a day, it's not optimal. If you can store more, it would be a good idea to do so. If you live in an apartment with no backyard hose from which to fill WaterBricks or 55-gallon drums to store in your basement or pantry, try to find every nook and cranny in your apartment where you can store some container and fill it with water. At least, equip yourself with a WaterBOB. Keep in mind, if you're storing dehydrated food, you'll have to store extra water for rehydration to prepare your food.

Cleanliness is not only important to stop the transmission of microorganisms but also provides a good boost to one's mood. If you're going to be in your SIRQ for any length of time, morale is going to be an important issue. If you're on your own well and you have backup power for the pump, nothing much should change. But if you're on city or town water, then you're going to need some options. For example, we have multiple solar shower bags from camping supply stores. These bags can be filled with up to 5 gallons of water, left in the sunlight until the temperature on the bag's thermometer reads a safe and comfortable temperature, and then gravity does the rest. Depending on your situation, you could put your solar shower bags in the sunlight on a deck or balcony within your perimeter. Then bring the bag inside, and hang it as high as possible from a hook in your bathroom over the shower. If you can't hang it high up, then hang it as high as possible, and get a shower chair or sit in the tub to make this work. Open the spray nozzle at the end of the tube hanging from the bag, and enjoy a hot shower with decent water pressure.

Even if the water isn't being pumped from the municipal source, there shouldn't be an issue with draining water down the tub. If that's a concern, or your bathroom isn't a suitable place to hang a solar shower bag, there are shower shelters, sometimes called privy shelters, that are designed to hang the solar shower bags. These shelters are large enough for one person to stand in comfortably and could be put outside on a deck, balcony, or yard, as you'll need to drain the water out of the bottom of the shelter. From personal experience, two of these solar shower bags are sufficient for our family (two adults, two children) each to get a good shower. Of course, rather than drain the water down the shower drain in your bathroom, or letting it drain below your deck, you could collect this water and use it to flush your toilet in the event that municipal water stopped running.

If water is at an absolute premium, another option is to stock up on baby wipes. This is a quick and easy way to freshen up, as well as to remove dirt and sweat. Baby wipes create trash, but they can be burned.

Dry shampoo is another option as well. Dry shampoo can be purchased, or natural dry shampoos can be made at home with all sorts of herbs and powders. You can get very fancy, using cosmetic clays, lavender, and rose powders, or even cocoa powder. You can also use a medicated powder, something like Gold Bond, which is mostly talc with menthol added. If you have an itchy scalp from not being able to shower the way you're used to, this can provide a lot of comfort while absorbing the excess oils from your hair. Just shake the powder onto the roots, work into the hair with your hands, just as if you were shampooing, and then brush out. Use a little at a time. You can always go back and powder an area again, but if you dump too much into your hair, you will get a sort of powdered wig look to it.

For those who would like to make an herbal dry shampoo, you can try this:

- ½ cup arrowroot (*Maranta arundinacea*)
- ¼ cup cosmetic clay
- ¼ cup baking soda
- 2 tablespoons oatstraw powder (*Avena sativa*)
- 1 tablespoon lavender flower powder
- 5 drops rosemary essential oil
- 5 drops lavender essential oil

Sift your dry ingredients together. To this, add in your essential oils, and blend well. If the oils begin to clump, use the back of a spoon to break up the clumps. Working quickly, transfer them to a bottle with a shaker top. Ingredients and packaging supplies can be found online from herbal suppliers, as well as on Amazon.

Soap is always better than hand sanitizer. But if you're running low on water, hand sanitizer is better than nothing. Most commercially made hand sanitizers contains triclosan, which has been linked to endocrine disorders and the creation of drug-resistant bacteria. If the claim is that a commercial gel is all-natural, it's likely alcohol based. The problem is that once you apply the gel to the skin, the alcohol begins to evaporate. Whatever the alcohol hasn't killed within two minutes won't be, unless there's another agent in the gel. Alcohol, even though it evaporates, is also tough on the skin.

If you would like to make some yourself, this is what I make for our bug-out bags and my emergency herbal medicine kit.

- ½ cup aloe vera gel
- 2 tablespoons witch hazel extract (*Hamamelis virginiana*)
- 80 drops lavender essential oil
- 50 drops rosalina essential oil
- 40 drops lemon essential oil
- 30 drops tea tree essential oil
- 20 drops thyme essential oil

Mix everything together in a bowl, and using a funnel or a cake decorating bag, fill a squeeze bottle with your natural hand sanitizer. Apply as you would any commercial hand sanitizer.

If you're using fresh aloe vera juice from a plant, you'll have to add some kind of preservative, most likely potassium sorbate, ascorbic acid, or citric acid. These are relatively easy to get from soap-making companies and herbal supply companies. If you buy all-natural aloe vera gel, it'll already have one or more of these preservatives in it. If you want to make something purely natural, then use aloe gel straight from the plant, and add the oils and witch hazel. Store in the fridge and use up within a week. It may last a little longer because of the essential oils, but there's no guarantee.

Waste Removal

This will be a major issue for anyone who currently relies on municipal waste removal services, such as trash removal and recycling programs. Waste removal also encompasses human wastes. If a pandemic hits an area so hard that people stop going to work to the extent that city trash trucks are no longer running, or at least are not running regularly, the same can be expected of municipal water department employees. This may lead to interruptions in the service and no running showers or flushing toilets.

You'll have to find ways to reduce your trash. Trash attracts rodents, and that's never good news. Here are some ideas to reduce your trash production.

- Reduce paper waste by turning paper trash into paper bricks, useful for starting fires in appropriate stoves and containers.
- Use cardboard boxes lined with plastic bags with holes for drainage, and use as a planter for growing food indoors.
- Cardboard can be used to stick in drafts from doors and windows, and cardboard installed at least one-quarter of an inch from the window should avoid issues with wicking moisture into the cardboard, and ultimately, disintegrating it.
- Cardboard boxes can be used to organize jars of pressure-canned meats and vegetables in your pantry.
- Vegetable scraps can be put in a compost pile or composted indoors with either a worm bin or Bokashi. Bokashi is a fermented bran product that uses microorganisms to compost vegetable, meat, and dairy products. It is a convenient method, but it requires that you stock up on the bran. Eventually, you will have to bury the Bokashi-composted material in soil to completely break down. Another good options is to feed kitchen scraps to chickens to reduce the need for commercial feed.
- If you have access to a yard or balcony where you can safely burn some of your trash, either in a fire pit or in a metal trash can, you can burn your trash. Try not to burn plastics.
- Reduce the amount of plastic trash you generate, and reuse plastics when you can, rather than create more piles of rodent-attracting trash. For example, use bread bags over your socks before you put your boots on. This creates a waterproof barrier that may have worn out on previously waterproofed items.

Human and pet waste must be disposed of properly, otherwise you run the risk of serious illness. If you're on a septic system, you should be OK. But if your septic system backs up, you may not be able to get anyone to come and service it, which would leave you with a yard saturated with human waste and potentially having it back up into your home. Make sure your septic system is operating as it should, and keep up with all regular maintenance.

If you're on a public sewer system, you should be OK unless the water stops flowing. If that happens, you still might be OK if you have water on hand that you can use for flushing. For example, if you wash your dishes in a rubber basin, or you collected the water from your solar shower, you can then use that gray water to flush the toilet.

If that doesn't work, however, what then? What if you have absolutely no gray water to flush your toilet: what options do you have? This is a critical decision because if you don't manage and dispose of your human waste properly, you risk serious, even life-threatening infections. When an entire community is improperly disposing of waste, this problem becomes compounded. Infections like E. coli would be very common, and if the circumstances were right, you could expect cholera as well.

A Special Note about Cholera

Cholera is typically found where there's poor sanitation. It may exist in the environment, in brackish water, like estuaries, or in raw shellfish. So, if you live near a coast, and part of your plan for feeding your family involves shellfish, be extra careful handling it and take care to cook it properly. Furthermore, if individuals infected with cholera don't dispose of their waste safely, the infection may spread rapidly through the water or soil. Consider what could happen if you don't bury infected human waste deep enough and stop at only a foot or two down. Think about what that soil may look like after a severe rainstorm. The infected material may rise to the top, spreading the bacteria, *Vibrio cholerae*, into backyards, sewers, streets, and so on.

For those who have a serious case of diarrhea from cholera, symptoms include severe watery diarrhea, vomiting, and leg cramps. In some rare cases, death can happen within hours. It's important to know about, but not worry excessively about. While cholera is a common disease to emerge after a disaster, and there have been cholera pandemics in the past, I didn't include it on the list of what might be the next great pandemic for a few reasons.

Cholera is more of an epidemic, localized concern. Cholera is spread by drinking water or eating food contaminated by *Vibrio cholerae*. In the United States, cholera outbreaks would most likely happen postdiaster, and would be caused by inadequate treatment of sewage contaminating the entire municipal water supply. This places cities at a unique risk.

It's not difficult to prevent cholera. Maintain your own clean source of water and don't eat contaminated food, especially raw shellfish. It's not difficult to treat most cases of cholera. Early treatment with oral rehydration salts has led to a mortality rate of 1 percent.[50]

Symptoms. According to CDC, for most people who become ill, 90–95 percent will have only minor symptoms. Only 5–10 percent of those who contract cholera will have serious symptoms.

Stay prepared. While nothing is impossible, and cholera outbreaks are likely to happen after any disaster, I cannot see it becoming the disaster. The worst this might be is an epidemic, until the area sorted out its sanitation problem. For an individual or group, this is something to prepare for by securing your perimeter, having your own source of water or your own water storage, having your own food storage, and stocking up on oral rehydration salts. There are some commercially available packets with decent flavorings, like lemon, which really help encourage children to drink them. Or you can make DIY oral rehydration salts at home with some simple ingredients.

- 6 tablespoons sugar
- ½ level teaspoon salt
- 1 liter or 5 cups water
- Optional flavorings: small amounts of unsweetened Kool-Aid powder, Jell-O powder, apple, or orange juice.

Mix these ingredients together, and take a sip every five minutes until urination becomes normal. This would end up being about 3 quarts to 3 liters per day. This should be continued until the diarrhea symptoms cease.[51]

The herbal perspective. Herbs that help relieve diarrhea can be helpful for the symptoms, but I don't know of any specific herb clearly effective against *Vibrio cholerae*. These might include oak (*Quercus spp.*) bark, red raspberry leaf (*Rubus idaeus*), peppermint leaf, and Oregon grape root (or other berberine-containing herb). I would make a tincture out of Amur cork tree (*Phellodendron amurense*) instead of Oregon grape

---

50 http://www.cdc.gov/cholera/general.
51 http://rehydrate.org/faq/how-to-prepare-ors.htm.

root for the berberine because the cork tree is an invasive to my area, which is on the East Coast. Chaparral or algerita might be options if you live in the western or southern United States. Barberry and coptis are also options. Please avoid goldenseal, as it's endangered in the wild.

Back to the question of what to do when you can't store water to flush your toilet: the best option I have found are 5-gallon buckets with a snap-on toilet seat and lid. Luggable Loo is a company that makes the snap-on toilet seat. If you don't have any 5-gallon buckets available, Luggable Loo also sells a combination of 5-gallon bucket and lid. Some people line this with a trash bag and proceed to use the toilet. This will leave a smell and allow liquid to build up in the bag. If the bag has tears, you may have waste leaking into your bucket.

For one of our practice bug outs at our BOL, we tested a different setup. We used the snap-on lid with some of our existing 5-gallon buckets, and put a layer of cat litter at the bottom. You could use sawdust instead if you had enough on hand. We used a product called Feline Pine. The same product is available for horses at a much lower price, making it ideal to stock up on a few bags. After every time the toilet was used, more litter was added to the bucket to cover the "deposit." The litter absorbed the liquid and helped cover the odor of both liquid and solid waste. When the bucket was about two-thirds full, we put the original lid back on, sealing any odor until we had an opportunity to dump the bucket into a designated location. The bucket dumped easily and was far less messy than the various portable toilets we tested.

The next most convenient portable toilet was the Thetford Porta Potti. This was the easiest to empty with the least amount of mess of any toilet we tested that also used water in its system. It uses very little water and is the most like a regular flush toilet most people have in their homes. If you have the option of digging a deep hole and dumping, and you have a little gray water to spare for flushing, this may be more familiar to people than using a sawdust or kitty litter toilet. And if you have small children who may be learning to use a toilet, this may be the least intimidating option.

Energy

I'm referring to ways to keep warm in cold weather, keep cool in hot weather, cook your food, and ideally have some power in the event that electrical service becomes unreliable. But keep in mind that having power can also make you a target. A line of smoke from a chimney may draw the attention of people who want to get warm. A lighted apartment in a dark city will stick out like a sore thumb. Having a backup generator is great to keep a refrigerator running, but the noise is a tell-tale sign that you have more than what others have. Even the smell of food being cooked on a backyard grill can draw unwanted attention.

I'm not saying not to have solar panels or a generator or a wood stove. I would never tell someone not to grill up some burgers and dogs for the family. Those are all great options in the right conditions. Perhaps you live in area where you know your neighbors and can talk to them about getting their own backup power sources and even neighborhood security.

Certainly, if you have solar panels, ceiling fans, a fire pit grill, and a wood stove, life is going to be much more comfortable. If everyone around you has a grill or a wood stove, those things may not stand out much. But if you have concerns over security, or live somewhere that these comforts may not be typical, you might want to consider some other options.

Heat comes to mind first for me, since I live in New England. Heat is usually provided by gas, electricity, oil burner, wood stove, pellet stove, or perhaps masonry stove. While many homes have fireplaces, they're not efficient for heating, as they cause significant drafts. Also, if you haven't had your chimney cleaned, as many people forget to do, you could easily start a house fire.

Gas-heated homes with old systems may be fine, but the newer systems rely on electricity to get them started. So if you lose electrical power, you may lose heat, even if you heat with gas. You would also lose your flame on a gas stove as well. Oil delivery would not be ideal if you're attempting to maintain the integrity of your perimeter.

Wood stoves would send a trail of smoke into the air, announcing your comfort. However, depending on where you live, wood stoves may be so commonplace that it's a nonissue. Masonry stoves and rocket mass heaters work on the same principles. They both offer clean burns, producing very little smoke. Masonry stoves are large and expensive, however, and rocket mass heaters are generally not permitted by homeowner's insurance and won't pass inspection in any major metropolitan area in the United States. For those in city apartments, something like a small propane heater may work. The type we have has an automatic shutoff in case of any gas leak. We also have a small, portable camping stove that runs on nothing more than sticks. It's also capable of generating electrical power and charging items like cell phones and laptops.

Having rechargeable communications devices, like a cell phone, tablet, laptop, and radios can keep you up-to-date on what is happening around your area and around the world with the current pandemic and any other major news.

Financial Preparedness

This is the one area that most people neglect in their preparedness plan. One of the biggest excuses people have for ignoring financial preparedness is that you can't eat money. Variations on this include "you can't eat gold" and "you can't eat silver." I suppose you can't eat an investment portfolio either. I find this mind-set shortsighted. If you don't plan for your financial needs, you may well come out of this disaster with nothing. In fact, you may not come out of it at all.

The biggest thing that will keep you and your family from bugging out in time is the ability to take leave from work. If you're dependent on your job, and you have a mortgage, auto loan, student loan, and credit card debts, odds are you will not make the call to get out of dodge soon enough. There will be nagging doubt, is it really time to bug out? Is this too soon? What if we bug out and it turns out to be nothing?

Everyone's situation is different, and money can trigger difficult emotions. But you must take an honest look at your finances and do a budget. Just as building up food storage can seem overwhelming at times, building up a nest egg and paying off debt can feel overwhelming at first. And just as there's no secret to building up food storage, there's no secret to building your savings and getting out of debt. Take it in small steps, focus on smaller goals first, and keep the ball rolling. Next thing you know, you'll have the ability to walk away from a job knowing that you can meet all of your bills for an extended period of time.

This kind of statement generally meets with skepticism. Come up with small, doable goals, and eventually you'll find that you've made impressive strides toward financial independence. But you must start with a budget. Most of the people I know who fight jumping into financial preparedness with both feet resist this first step. You cannot know where you can save money, where you're wasting money, or if your debts have exceeding your income, without doing a budget.

If your income is less than your expenses, unlike our government, you cannot just print more money. If you're stuck financially, maybe one of the suggestions below might help:

- Sell your used books on Amazon.
- Sell your used clothes at a local consignment shop or on eBay.
- Teach a class in something you know about (soap making, piano lessons, beading, carving, home canning, etc.)
- Sell your garden produce, honey, maple syrup, baked goods, and so forth, at your local farmer's market.
- If you're crafty, open an Etsy shop.
- If you have the skills, take in alterations and sew for special occasions.
- Check out any of the free financial resources online, like Dave Ramsey's Debt Snowball.
- Make use of financial planning books specifically written with preppers in mind, such as Jim Cobb's book, *The Prepper's Financial Guide: Strategies to Invest, Stockpile, and Build Security for Today and the Post-Collapse Marketplace*.

If you do open your own business, keep your overhead low and focus on income-generating activities. It's easy to get caught up in this or that aspect of one's business, especially the parts we enjoy the most. But they must generate an income. If you find that you're spending far too much time on social media, or creating lots of content that you then shy away from promoting, you're just going to waste a lot of time and effort. Keep it simple.

Another possible option is working from home. If your job is such that it can be done online from home, perhaps it would be worth approaching your boss and asking whether he or she has ever considered continuity of operations in case of emergency, and how it would benefit the company to have key operations handled from home. It could be any emergency, from severe weather to a severe flu epidemic, which could affect efficiency. If you can demonstrate the financial benefits of having an emergency plan, you might have the option of having uninterrupted income for the duration of your SIRQ.

Banking during emergencies is always a bit risky. A quick look at what has happened in Greece and the "bank holiday" and likely "bail-ins" is enough to unnerve anyone. But if you can secure an income by working from home, having direct deposit, and using online banking, you should be able to maintain your current lifestyle for an extended period of time, without risking infection to you or your family.

Medical Preparedness

While this entire book is about illnesses and health, and how to avoid getting sick, this barely scratches the surface when it comes to medical preparedness. Consider that pandemics are generally long-term emergencies and hospitals are often overwhelmed by an immense flow of sick people trying to be seen for treatment. This means that other people with other illnesses, whether chronic or acute, probably won't be able to get the care they need.

What will you do if someone needs assistance with a birth during this crisis? Could you care for a laceration that was bleeding profusely? What would you do if someone in your group suffered a serious burn? As we learned from the Ebola outbreak in West Africa, often it isn't the pandemic disease that gets you, but some other medical emergency that comes up with no health professionals and no facilities available for treatment.

This is why you must designate someone in your group as the medic. This is the person who will be the go-to person if people catch a cold, sprain an ankle, suddenly find themselves with swollen joints for no apparent reason, or feel like they're having a heart attack. The medic will be responsible for maintaining what amounts to medical records for the group, understands what their base level of health is when the SIRQ began, monitors chronic conditions, helps improve them, and is there to respond in an emergency. The group's medic will oversee the reentry of any group member who had to leave the safety of the perimeter and is the individual responsible for anyone in quarantine before joining your group and anyone who may find themselves in isolation if they fall ill.

While your group may not be blessed with having a physician in your ranks, there's a lot of reliable information out there that we can use to get us through emergencies. There's a wealth of information available on specific illnesses on websites maintained by WHO and CDC. You can also sign up for the Center for Infectious Disease Research and Policy free e-mail newsletter. Pubmed.gov is a website that catalogs abstracts of published studies, many of which have links to the full study, often available as free PDFs, or links to where the study can be purchased.

Several doctors and medical professionals have put their educational hats on to help the public prepare for disasters. They have websites, books, online courses, DVDs, Facebook groups where you can interact with them and ask questions, and all manner of media to help you get better prepared to handle medical emergencies during a disaster. Sources from the modern medical world who stand out in this field are:

- Dr. James Hubbard, also known as the Survival Doctor, has written several practical books on burns, first aid, and the ingenious use of duct tape in medical emergencies. His website is loaded with useful information, and he offers an online course for when medical help is delayed and you suddenly become the first responder. Hubbard has a calm and clear way of laying out emergency medical information and is a fabulous resource for those who want to be more medically knowledgeable and prepared. His website is www.TheSurvivalDoctor.com.

- Dr. Joe Alton and Nurse Amy Alton of Doom and Bloom have books, an information-rich website, YouTube videos, DVDs, and a weekly podcast. They travel all over the United States to teach medical skills that will be most useful postdisaster. The Doom and Bloom team also has a board game specifically about surviving in a postpandemic disaster, which might be the perfect way to introduce family and friends to the concept and importance of preparing for a pandemic. Their website is www.DoomAndBloom.net.

- Former combat medic Chuck Hudson of The Medic Shack teaches his Battlefield Medic course in the New Mexico and Arizona area. Chuck says about his courses: "Where many survivalists can teach you to put holes in other people, I teach you how to patch them back up again." His courses are unique, testing your ability to get to injured people, triage, and rescue under hostile conditions, and also teaching advanced hands-on skills for when no other higher form of medical care is coming. Chuck and I cohost a weekly podcast exploring hypothetical postdisaster scenarios with both biomedicine and herbal medicine. Look for Chuck's upcoming courses and his "Tip of the week" on his website, www.TheMedicShack.net.

From outside the medical field, there's my website, www.Herbal Prepper.com, offering online classes, announcements on local courses, and loads of herbal articles. My first book, *Prepper's Natural Medicine: Lifesaving Herbs, Essential Oils, and Natural Remedies for When There Is No Doctor* is the next best option if you can't take one of my herbal courses in person or online. This covers a range of herbal skills specifically for the everyday illnesses, as well as the emergency situations that may occur during a long-term crisis.

For a unique experience where you can be fully immersed in postdisaster skills training, check out The Human Path, run by an herbalist and former Special Forces combat medic, Sam Coffman. If you're serious about functioning as your group's medic, especially in case of pandemics, this school provides a hands-on, in-the-field learning experience on communications, water filtration, herbal medicine, wilderness first aid certification, and postdisaster engineering, just to name a few. There are many survival schools around, but The Human Path goes further by not only teaching you how to survive catastrophes but also how to rebuild afterward. There are tons of off-grid and sustainability courses as well. The school is located in San Antonio, Texas, and offers everything a prepper, survivalist, or herbalist could want to take their game to the next level. Take a moment to visit his school's website at www.TheHumanPath.com.

Medical Equipment

If you're preparing to care for people's health when there's no doctor, you should have on hand, and know how to use, some basic medical equipment. In addition to keeping medical records, you should also know how to take vital signs. Vital signs are measurements of the body's basic functions, and these measurements give us our first clues into how healthy a person is, as well as what might be ailing the patient.

Vital sign measurements include:

- Body temperature
- Pulse rate
- Respiration rate
- Blood pressure

While not technically a "vital sign," a blood pressure reading is usually done at this time. I included it in the list for the sake of completion, and to help people remember that this is the time to get a blood pressure reading.

Each of these measurements have a range that's considered normal. Be prepared to see variation, but readings outside these ranges generally indicate some kind of illness. Let's go through each measurement, how to record it, and what measurements outside the range of normal might mean.

Body Temperature. Average normal body temperature is 98.6°F (37°C). Normal body temperature ranges between 97.8°F (36.5°C) and 99°F (37.2°C). Body temperature is measured with a thermometer.

There's the classic glass thermometer, which contains mercury. These are reliable and do not require batteries. But they're easy to break, and the mercury inside is toxic. A mercury spill would create an environmental hazard, and no one needs that added problem in the middle of a SIRQ.

A temperature can be obtained from an oral, rectal, or axillary (armpit) reading with a traditional, glass thermometer. If you have a newer, digital thermometer, a temperature can be obtained more easily, faster, and cleaner via the ear or skin along the forehead. These thermometers do require a battery. But they can often scan quickly and don't present an environmental contamination risk if dropped. Always disinfect the thermometer between patients.

If a temperature falls outside the normal range, or very close to it, here are some things to keep in mind. If the body temperature is very low, for instance, 95°F (35°C), the patient is hypothermic. If the body temperature is only slightly lower than normal, or even on the border of normal at 97.8°F (36.5°C), and there hasn't been cold weather or other reason for the lower temperature, there may be a metabolic reason for it. Many of the body's metabolic functions are controlled by the thyroid gland, which is a butterfly-shaped gland located at your throat. A hypoactive (underactive) thyroid may be to blame for a slightly lower temperature. Conversely, if the temperature is elevated, and the weather has been ruled out as a possibility, a hyperactive (overactive) thyroid may be the cause. However, the most common reason for an elevated temperature is a fever. A fever is generally a sign alerting you that the body is fighting infection.

While the conventional wisdom has been to administer fever-reducing medications, a fever is one of the body's natural responses to infections. The body is raising its temperature to make it inhospitable to bacteria and viruses. If we interrupt the process, we may be prolonging the illness. Eventually the fever spikes and breaks, leaving the patient to sweat and cool down.

Pulse Rate. The pulse rate is the number of times the heart beats per minute. The pulse can tell us if the heartbeat is regular and strong, or if there's a potential problem. The normal pulse rate for adults is 60 to 100 per minute, depending on activity level. If your pulse is resting at 50 beats per minute, but you're an athlete with a strong cardiovascular system, that may be your personal normal. If you experience your pulse speed up dramatically to 100 just getting up from a chair, that's not normal.

The pulse rate is taken by placing your fingers over an artery, pressing it against a bony structure underneath, and counting the pulses. This may be done in seven different places on the body:

- Carotid artery (side of the neck)
- Brachial artery (inside elbow)
- Radial artery (thumb side of the wrist)
- Femoral artery (upper thigh)
- Popliteal artery (inner knee)
- Dorsalis pedis (top of foot, toward the middle of the body, above the edge of the arch)
- Posterior tibial artery (behind the ankle along the medial side)

The only way to get good at taking a pulse is to do it, and do it often, trying it out on as many people as possible. Use whichever pulse you need to, though I almost always prefer to take the radial pulse at the wrist. To measure the pulse rate, count how many times the heart beats in fifteen seconds. Then multiply by four.

How to Take a Blood Pressure Reading. There are several ways you can do this. There are easy cuffs that are battery operated that you can strap onto someone's wrist, and it will provide you a quick and easy read out. A proper reading, however, is usually done with a blood pressure cuff, also called a sphygmomanometer, and a stethoscope. There are pros and cons to both, such as if the battery runs out on the wrist cuff, then you're out of luck. You won't be able to take any more readings. The wrist readings may not be entirely precise, but should get you pretty close. A more accurate reading can be done with the blood pressure cuff and stethoscope, but if you're not accustomed to using one, you can easily miss hearing the clicks or miscount the heart beats. If you're going to take your readings manually, make sure to practice taking readings frequently. Practice all your skills frequently. During an emergency isn't the time to begin learning.

Since we're talking about emergencies, be aware that stress raises blood pressure. If possible, allow the patient to calm down before taking the reading. Otherwise, you'll get an artificially high reading. Always use an appropriately sized arm cuff. Attempting to read a blood pressure with a regular cuff when the person needs an extra-large cuff will guarantee an artificially high reading.

Follow these steps to take a blood pressure reading:

- Wrap the blood pressure cuff around the upper arm, about 1 inch above the inside of the elbow, also called the antecubital fossa.
- Take the bell of the stethoscope, and position it just under the cuff, slightly higher than the inner elbow. Apply light pressure. You should find the brachial artery easily this way.
- Rapidly inflate the cuff with the hand pump until you see the hand indicate 180.
- Slowly release a little air.
- While the air releases, listen for a clicking or a knocking sound. You will see a simultaneous pulsing of the hand on your sphygmomanometer with each click. If the environment is too loud, or your stethoscope is in backward (that happens easier than one might think), you may have trouble hearing the clicks. But you'll see them on the dial readout.
- The number where those clicks start is the systolic blood pressure (top number).
- The number where those clicks stop is the diastolic blood pressure (bottom number).

There are ranges of blood pressures, from hypotensive (low), ideal, prehypertensive, and hypertensive (high).

- 90/60 or lower indicates low blood pressure.
- More than 90/60 and less than 120/80 is considered ideal.
- More than 120/80 and less than 140/90 indicates OK, but borderline high blood pressure.
- 140/90 indicates high blood pressure.

Oxygen. Oxygen is part of the standard treatments for several of the illnesses explored in this book. Oxygen may also be helpful in cardiac events. Emergency oxygen units are available for first aid without a prescription. The kits include three types of equipment. There's the oxygen cylinder (tank), a pressure regulator with a flowmeter to control the airflow, and a delivery device, such as prongs (nasal cannulas) or a rebreather mask.

These kits run between $100 and $500, and come with either prongs that are inserted into the nasal cavities or a rebreather mask. Instructions come with every kit. Take the time to look over the instructions and understand how to operate your kit if the need should arise. Please use caution when handling oxygen tanks and using oxygen. These tanks can do serious damage when mishandled. Keep an eye on the pressure gauge, do not use around open flames, and follow every safety precaution included in your kit.

The Importance of Renewable Medicine

Pharmacies, along with grocery stores and hospitals, are among the first resources to be raided and picked clean during a disaster. When that disaster also involves a pandemic, going to the pharmacy may mean risking infection. I suggest that herbs and other natural substances, such as honey, clay, and activated charcoal, can fill in much if not all of the gap left by people who cannot get a refill on their normal prescriptions.

I cannot stress enough the importance of dealing with chronic illnesses before a pandemic illness shows up at your doorstep. Any improvement at all improves your chances of survival. That being said, there will be many people dependent on maintenance medications for diabetes, hypertension, cholesterol, arthritis, and psychological issues who will be suddenly cut off from their drugs. Many of them will not survive. There are also acute conditions, such as a broken leg, a gun shot wound, or a urinary tract infection.

You need a plan to handle both chronic and acute conditions, not just the particular pandemic that might or might not make it to your doorstep. My suggestion is to learn about herbal medicine. Herbal medicine is effective, under your control, affordable, and can be grown right in your own backyard, on your homestead, or even in a few pots in a sunny window. If you're into guerrilla gardening you can plant medicinal herbs in some of the most unlikely places. Most other people would never notice the plants, but you know where they are and what they do.

My herbal supplies include tinctures, glycerites, herbal vinegars, salves, infused oils, honey, activated charcoal, kaolin and bentonite clay, essential oils, carrier oils, teas, and poultices. The specific remedies you may want to keep on hand will be determined by the kinds of illnesses and injuries you expect to see. If you're diabetic, you may want to stock up on *Gymnema sylvestre* or grow fenugreek (*Trigonella foenum-graecum*) or goat's rue (*Galega officinalis*). Goat's rue is the herbal origin of the active ingredients in metformin, galegine, and guanidine. If you have a heart condition, you might want to grow a hawthorn tree and motherwort (*Leonurus cardiaca*) in your herbal garden. I would also want to keep around some general things, like an herbal antibiotic formula and an herbal antiviral formula, something to fight fungal infections and stop bleeding.

The Prepper's Ultimate Pandemic Preparedness Kit

The following is what I currently keep in my large kit, which takes up several plastic totes. This would be what I take with me on a practice bug out where I set up a designated "infirmary" area. This is just an outline, to give you an idea of what to stock up on. If the herbs or terms are unfamiliar to you, I strongly recommend that you find an herbal class near you, or check out the resource section for books and online training.

PREPAREDNESS KIT	
CATEGORY	**ITEMS**
Personal protective equipment (PPE)	• Gloves • Face mask • Large trash bag and duct tape • Safety goggles • Tyvek suit or garbage bags and duct tape
Medical equipment and supplies	• Blood pressure cuff (sphygmomanometer) • Stethoscope • Emergency oxygen • Pulse oximeter • Portable defibrillator • Otoscope • Flashlight • Tongue depressors • Alcohol wipes • Snips • Razor blades or scalpel • Forceps • Tweezers • Oral rehydration salts (ORS) • Hot water bottle • Enema bag and hose • Douche • Probiotic tablets • Water
Bandaging	• Gauze pads • Tape • Vet tape • Ace bandage • Butterfly bandages, Steri-Strips, or duct tape
Bleeding	• QuikClot (kaolin clay) • Postpartum pads • Tampons • Wound powder formula including yarrow • Yarrow tincture • Shepherd's purse tincture • Tourniquet or Israeli bandage
Wound wash/soak ingredients	Hibiclens (skin cleanser and antiseptic) or astringent, anti-inflammatory, and anti-infective herbs such as: • Oak • Calendula • Calendula water/hydrosol • Chaparral • Lavender water/hydrosol • Oregon grape root • Rose water/hydrosol • White willow • Witch hazel • Yarrow
Activated charcoal	Good for: • Accidental poisoning • Food poisoning • Wound care • Spider and snake bites • *Staphylococcus aureus* infections
Bentonite clay	Good for: • Ringworm • Boils (staph infections where skin is intact) • Poison ivy or oak

PREPAREDNESS KIT

CATEGORY	ITEMS	
Honey	Good for: • Burns • Puncture wounds • Deep wounds • *Staphylococcus aureas* infections	• Soothing to tissues • Sore throats • Ingredient in syrups
Alliderm: Garlic	This seems like a useful product to keep in a first aid or trauma kit, as the allicin in garlic has a short half-life. That half-life is about six days, and longer if preserved with a combination of alcohol and water, such as in a tincture. Using an alcohol-based tincture on an open wound would sting, at the very least. Having this gel on hand would be very useful. But you could also apply a fresh solution of crushed garlic in water or garlic honey to the infection.	
Dry Herbs: Singles	• Aloe • Comfrey	• Nettle • Peppermint tea bags
Dry Herbs: Formulas	Respiratory tea: Mix ingredients below, fill a zip-top bag for your kit, store the rest in a sealed mylar bag with an oxygen absorber or a vacuum sealed mason jar. • 2 cups hyssop • 1½ cups mullein leaves • 1½ cups slippery elm • 1 cup elecampane	• ½ cup coltsfoot • ½ cup peppermint • ½ cup licorice • ½ cup cloves
Salves	Good for: • Muscle and nerve pain (cayenne and St. John's wort) • Sprains, bruises, and joint pain (arnica and comfrey) • Bites and blisters (plantain and comfrey) Infuse herbs of choice into olive oil. Use 1 cup of oil to 2 tablespoons or 1 ounce of beeswax to make the salve. Melt the beeswax into the salve. Once the pastilles are gone, pour into containers and let cool.	
Wound powder	• 1 part chaparral • 1 part yarrow • 1 part calendula	• 1 part usnea • 1 part kaolin clay

PREPAREDNESS KIT	
CATEGORY	**ITEMS**
Tinctures: Singles	Good for: • Lobelia: muscle relaxant, antispasmodic • Echinacea: anti-infective, immune support • Spilanthes: mouth pain and infections • Ma Huang, aka ephedra, or mormon tea: allergic reactions • Nettle (leaf and seed): antihistamine, analgesic, diuretic; seed is an adaptogen • Rhodiola: mood enhancement, anti-anxiety, no drowsiness
Tinctures: Formulas	Good for: • Pain: major (3 parts California poppy, 2 parts corydalis, 1 part Jamaican dogwood) • Pain: minor–average (1 part white willow or meadowsweet, 1 part Solomon's seal, 1 part codonopsis) • Anti-anxiety/Calming glycerite (3 parts lemon balm, 1 part passionflower) • Sedative formula (4 parts American skullcap, 2 parts valerian, 1 part Jamaican dogwood) • Antibiotic formula (4 parts *Sida acuta*, 4 parts *Artemisia annua* or Sweet Annie, 3 parts echinacea, 2 parts juniper berry, 2 parts usnea, 2 parts garlic) • Antiviral formula (3 parts Chinese skullcap, 3 parts red sage, 3 parts dong quai, 2 parts elderberry, 2 parts echinacea, 1 part ginger, 1 part licorice) • Antifungal formula (6 parts calendula, 2 parts Oregon grape root, 1 part black walnut) • Antiprotozoan formula (1 part wormwood, 1 part black walnut, 1 part garlic, 1 part horseradish, 1 part milk thistle, 1 part cloves, 1 part thyme, 1 part berberine-containing herb of your choice) • Anti-inflammatory formula (3 parts yerba mansa, 1 part turmeric) • Anti-inflammatory/Antispasmodic formula (1 part black cohosh, 1 part white willow or meadowsweet, 1 part cayenne, 1 part lobelia) *Could be made into a salve instead* • Allergy formula (1 part Ma huang, 1 part nettle leaf) • Liver formula (6 parts milk thistle, 3 parts burdock, 1 part dandelion) • Cardiac formula (6 parts hawthorn berries, 4 parts motherwort, 2 parts garlic, 1 part cayenne or red pepper flakes)

Many things could be added to this list, but this is intended as a starting point, not an end point. Herbal formulas for pregnant women, diabetics, children, and any other category you can think of could be added here if it will affect you.

Pandemics will happen. When, where, what, for how long, and how bad will it be? I don't know. No one knows. What I do know, however, is that being prepared means that you and your loved ones stand a greater chance of surviving something as devastating and as drawn out as a pandemic.

In the meantime, enjoy learning new skills. Enjoy learning how to can and dehydrate food. Enjoy your time in the garden growing both food and medicine. Enjoy practicing a bug out: treat it as a family camping trip. Prepping has always seemed to me more like having hundreds of practical hobbies. Enjoy prepping for a pandemic!

Conclusion

After all the consideration of scary, deadly, infectious diseases in this book, the conclusion I have come to, and that I hope readers have also come to, is twofold: that we have options and that we are fortunate.

- We have the option to take a proactive role in securing our future well-being.
- We have the option to improve our health now, improve chronic illness and fitness, and reduce our overall risk during any crisis.
- We have the option to decide that medical and financial preparedness matter for long-term security, and to act on that decision.
- We are fortunate to have access, either in local stores or online from specialty suppliers, to preparedness, medical, herbal, and food supplies that generations past and those living in much poorer parts of the world couldn't imagine.
- We are fortunate that a deadly pandemic has not broken out in the United States in recent memory.

We don't prepare for such things as pandemics and other potential life-as-we-know-it altering events because we're fearful or negative. We prepare because we have hope, an expectation that in the end, these disasters are survivable. We prepare because we have a drive to survive, and even to thrive, no matter what.

Resources

Recommended Reading

Aromatherapy

Essential Oil Safety: A Guide for Health Care Professionals, by Robert Tisserand and Rodney Young (Churchill Livingstone, 2013)

Herbal Books

The Book of Herbal Wisdom: Using Plants as Medicine, by Matthew Wood (North Atlantic Books, 1997)

Herbal Antibiotics: Natural Alternatives for Treating Drug-Resistant Bacteria, by Stephen Harrod Buhner (Storey Publishing, 2012)

Herbal Antivirals: Natural Remedies for Emerging and Resistant Viral Infections, by Stephen Harrod Buhner (Storey Publishing, 2013)

Herbal Healing for Women: Simple Home Remedies for Women of All Ages, by Rosemary Gladstar (Simon and Schuster, 1993)

The Herbal Medicine-Maker's Handbook: A Home Manual, by James Green (Crossing Press, 2000)

Medical Herbalism: The Science and Practice of Herbal Medicine, by David Hoffman (Healing Arts Press, 2003)

Nutritional Herbology: A Reference Guide to Herbs, by Mark Pedersen (Whitman Publications, 2012)

The Practice of Traditional Western Herbalism: Basic Doctrine, Energetics, and Classification, by Matthew Wood (North Atlantic Books, 2013)

Principles and Practice of Phytotherapy: Modern Herbal Medicine, 2nd ed., by Kerry Bone and Simon Mills (Churchill Livingstone, 2013)

Holistic Health

Holistic Anatomy: An Integrative Guide to the Human Body, by Pip Waller (North Atlantic Books, 2010)

Medical Preparedness First Aid

Living Ready Pocket Manual—First Aid: Fundamentals for Survival, by James Hubbard, MD, MPH (Living Ready, 2013)

The Survival Handbook: A Guide for When Help Is Not on the Way, by Joe Alton and Amy Alton (Doom and Bloom, 2013)

Midwifery and Women's Health

Birth Emergency Skills Training: Manual for Out-of-Hospital Midwives, by Bonnie Gruenberg (Birth Guru Publications, 2008)

A Book for Midwives: Care for Pregnancy, Birth, and Women's Health, by Susan Klein (Hesperian Foundation, 2013)

Heart and Hands: A Midwife's Guide to Pregnancy and Birth, by Elizabeth Davis (Celestial Arts, 2004)

Holistic Midwifery: A Comprehensive Textbook for Midwives in Homebirth Practice, vol. 1: Care during Pregnancy, by Anne Frye (Labrys Press, 2010)

Taking Charge of Your Fertility: The Definitive Guide to Natural Birth Control, Pregnancy Achievement, and Reproductive Health, by Toni Weschler (William Morrow Paperbacks, 2006)

Nutrition and Fermented Foods

Nourishing Traditions: The Cookbook That Challenges Politically Correct Nutrition and the Diet Dictocrats, by Sally Fallon and Mary Enig (Newtrends Publishing, Inc., 2010)

Nutritional Herbology: A Reference Guide to Herbs, by Mark Pedersen (Whitman Publications, 2012)

Wild Fermentation: The Flavor, Nutrition, and Craft of Live-Culture Foods, by Sandor Ellix Katz and Sally Fallon (Chelsea Green Publishing, 2003)

Preparedness Books

The Prepper's Blueprint: The Step-by-Step Guide to Help You through Any Disaster, by Tess Pennington and Daisy Luther (CreateSpace, 2014)

Prepper's Financial Guide: Strategies to Invest, Stockpile, and Build Security for Today and the Post-Collapse Marketplace, by Jim Cobb (Ulysses Press, 2015)

Prepper's Home Defense: Security Strategies to Protect Your Family by Any Means Necessary, by Jim Cobb (Ulysses Press, 2012)

The Prepper's Water Survival Guide: Harvest, Treat, and Store Your Most Vital Resource, by Daisy Luther (Ulysses Press, 2015)

Websites

Education/Research

Doom and Bloom Survival Medicine, www.doomandbloom.net

The Enchanter's Green, enchantersgreen.com

Henriette's Herbal Page, www.henriettes-herb.com

Herbal Prepper, www.herbalprepper.com

The Human Path, thehumanpath.net

The Medic Shack, www.themedicshack.net

A Modern Herbal by Mrs. M. Grieve, www.botanical.com

Prepper Broadcasting Network, www.prepperbroadcasting.com

PubMed, www.ncbi.nlm.nih.gov/pubmed

Robin Rose Bennett, Herbalist, www.robinrosebennett.com

Sage Mountain Herbal Education Center, www.sagemountain.com

Southwest School of Botanical Medicine, www.swsbm.com

The Survival Doctor, www.thesurvivaldoctor.com

Organizations

American Herbalists Guild, www.americanherbalistsguild.com
Free Fire Cider, freefirecider.com
National Health Freedom Coalition, www.nationalhealthfreedom.org

Publications

The Essential Herbal magazine, www.essentialherbal.com
Plant Healer magazine, www.planthealermagazine.com
Prepare Magazine, www.preparemag.com

Seeds

Strictly Medicinal Seeds, www.strictlymedicinalseeds.com
Sand Mountain Herbs, www.sandmountainherbs.com

Suppliers

Organic Alcohol Company, organicalcohol.com
Bulk Herb Store, www.bulkherbstore.com
Cultures for Health, www.culturesforhealth.com
Jean's Greens, www.jeansgreens.com
Mountain Rose Herbs, www.mountainroseherbs.com
SKS Bottle and Packaging, www.sks-bottle.com
Soaper's Choice, www.soaperschoice.com

Index

Hubbard, James, and medical preparedness, 160–61
Hudson, Chuck, and medic courses, 161
Human error, and release of pathogens, 108–109
Human immunodeficiency virus (HIV), 130–31
The Human Path (postdisaster skills training), 161–62
Human waste. *See* Waste
The Humanure Handbook, 41

Incinerating toilets, and waste disposal, 40, 41
Influenza, 49, 50–60; conventional responses, 55–56; natural/herbal responses, 56–60; pandemics, 51–52; risk factors, 53–54; symptoms, 54–55, 103; threat assessment points, 50; transmission, 55; treatment responses, 55–60; types, 51
Insect-to-person disease transmission, 34: and bunyaviruses, 96; deterrence, 144; and ebola, 99; and flaviviruses, 98, 99; and plague, 33, 114, 115; and Powassan, 23; and "The Surprise," 123; and VHFs, 100
Intravenous fluids, at home, 101–102, 103
Ionizing diffusers, 84
Isolation, and disease prevention, 35–36; vs. quarantine, 142–43
Ivory Coast virus, 98. *See also* Ebola (2014); Filoviruses

Jenkins, Joseph, 41

K. pneumoniae, 75
Kitty litter toilets, 155
Klain, Ron ("Ebola czar"), 17, 19

Lassa virus, 96. *See also* Arenaviruses
Latent tuberculosis, 60–61
Listeria, 78
Livestock, and antibiotics, 29
Luggable Loo, 155
Lujo virus, 96. *See also* Arenaviruses

Machupo virus, 96. *See also* Arenaviruses
Maintenance drugs, 29
Marburgvirus, 97–98. *See also* Filoviruses
Marigolds, as bug repellent, 144
Marseilles Vinegar (homemade), 120–21
Masks. *See* Face masks
MDR efflux pump, 30
Measles, 125–27
Medical equipment, and SIRQ, 162–66
Medical preparedness, and SIRQ, 159–66
MERS. *See* Middle East respiratory syndrome
Methicillin, 74–75
Mice. *See* Rodents
Middle East respiratory syndrome (MERS), 4–5, 23, 44–45, 89–91. *See also* Coronaviruses
Mint. *See* Peppermint
Monkeys, as "bushmeat," 23, 99
Morale, and SIRQ, 149
Mosquitos. *See* Insect-to-person disease transmission

Acknowledgments

A most heartfelt and grateful thank you to my dear husband, Eddie. I'm truly fortunate to have such a supportive, generous, and genuinely kind man as my partner. Whenever I needed anything, you were right there. And when I was locked away for hours writing, you were understanding and encouraging. Thank you. Without you, this book could not have happened.

To my children, I am so proud of you both. You have challenged a spontaneous, artistic spirit like me to value my time, set boundaries, and embrace organization. I'm thrilled that you both have developed a love of reading and books and plants. You inspire me every day.

A huge thank-you goes to Chuck Hudson for allowing me to pick his brain, and for filling in the blanks in some areas in which I am not well versed. I thank you also for your humor. However, I can no longer look at cinnamon the same way again. Your friendship is appreciated more than you realize.

Thank you to all the listeners at Prepper Broadcasting and at The Survival Circle. The questions that came to my inbox or popped up in the chat room are what prompted this book. Doing these broadcasts have put me in touch with so many wonderful people, and I am grateful for each one of you.

A major thank you to my editor, Casie Vogel, who was able to help put organization to the massive collection of data that was the original manuscript. I greatly appreciate your ideas and guidance that turned this overwhelming collection of research notes into a usable and accessible guide.

Thank you to Ulysses Press for the opportunity to write this book, and its entire team of professionals for turning this book into a reality. I'm filled with gratitude for having had this experience.

Thank you to Tess Pennington for writing the foreword to this book. I'm a huge fan of your books and your blog. I appreciate your words here and admire the work you do for the prepping community. You are truly a class act. Thank you for all your support.

I also have to thank my friend and fellow Ulysses Press author, Daisy Luther. Our chats have kept me sane and laughing no matter how stressful the juggling act between work and family got this past year. You crack me up, you have such a beautiful heart, and I'm so glad to have found another kindred spirit in the prepping world.

About the Author

Cat Ellis is a practicing herbalist and dedicated prepper. Her love of herbs began in the 1990s when herbs helped her recover from the flu. Cat now sees clients and teaches herbal medicine through her private practice, Herbwyfery. She is also a massage therapist, certified in MotherMassage™, and a member of the American Herbalists Guild.

Economic pressures and a desire for greater freedoms sparked Cat's interest in survivalism and homesteading in 2008. She describes prepping as having "hundreds of practical hobbies," like gardening, canning, and self-defense. For Cat, being prepared brings both peace of mind and personal satisfaction.

Cat's love of herbal medicine merged with her love of prepping, resulting in her website, www.HerbalPrepper.com. She is the author of *Prepper's Natural Medicine: Lifesaving Herbs, Essential Oils, and Natural Remedies for When There Is No Doctor*, and her articles have been published in PREPARE magazine. Cat has also ventured into the world of broadcasting, with two weekly, live, Internet radio shows. Cat hosts her own show, *Herbal Prepper Live*, on the Prepper Broadcasting Network, as well as cohosting *The Medic Shack*, on The Survival Circle Radio Network.